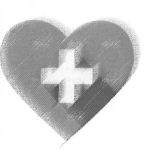

EMPATHY
STORIES
INSPIRE AND
ENLIGHTEN BUSY
CLINICIANS

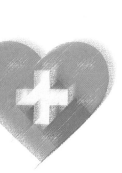

EMPATHY: REAL STORIES TO INSPIRE AND ENLIGHTEN BUSY CLINICIANS

Daniel E. Epner, MD, FACP

Professor
Department of Palliative, Rehabilitation, and Integrative Medicine
The University of Texas MD Anderson Cancer Center
Houston, Texas

NEW YORK   CHICAGO   SAN FRANCISCO   ATHENS
LONDON   MADRID   MEXICO CITY   MILAN
NEW DELHI   SINGAPORE   SYDNEY   TORONTO

Empathy: Real Stories to Inspire and Enlighten Busy Clinicians

1 2 3 4 5 6 7 8 9 LCR 27 26 25 24 23 22

ISBN 978-1-260-47341-4
MHID 1-260-47341-4

The editors were Jason Malley and Christina M. Thomas
The production supervisor was Richard Ruzycka.
Project management was provided by MPS Ltd.
The cover designer was W2 Design.
Cover Photo: Margeaux C. Epner, MD
This book is printed on acid-free paper.

Library of Congress Control Number: 2022930913

For Linda, Margeaux, and Eden, my sources
of light and inspiration

Contents

Contributors

Sujin Ann-Yi, PhD
Assistant Professor of Palliative, Rehabilitation, and Integrative Medicine
The University of Texas MD Anderson Cancer Center
Houston, Texas

Joseph Arthur, MBCHB
Associate Professor of Palliative, Rehabilitation, and Integrative Medicine
The University of Texas MD Anderson Cancer Center
Houston, Texas

Ahsan Azhar, MD
Assistant Professor of Palliative, Rehabilitation, and Integrative Medicine
The University of Texas MD Anderson Cancer Center
Houston, Texas

Eduardo Bruera, MD
Professor and Chair of Palliative, Rehabilitation, and Integrative Medicine
The University of Texas MD Anderson Cancer Center
Houston, Texas

Marvin O. Delgado Guay, MD
Associate Professor of Palliative, Rehabilitation, and Integrative Medicine
The University of Texas MD Anderson Cancer Center
Houston, Texas

Daniel E. Epner, MD, FACP
Professor of Palliative, Rehabilitation, and Integrative Medicine
The University of Texas MD Anderson Cancer Center
Houston, Texas

Linda C. Epner, MD
Associate Professor of Ophthalmology
Baylor College of Medicine
Houston, Texas

Michael Frumovitz, MD, MPH
Professor of Gynecological Oncology & Reproductive Medicine
Ad Interim Chief Patient Experience Officer
The University of Texas MD Anderson Cancer Center
Houston, Texas

Isabella C. Glitza Oliva, MD, PhD
Associate Professor of Melanoma Medical Oncology
The University of Texas MD Anderson Cancer Center
Houston, Texas

Bruno P. Granwehr, MD
Professor of Infectious Diseases
The University of Texas MD Anderson Cancer Center
Houston, Texas

Faye M. Johnson, MD, PhD
Professor of Thoracic-Head & Neck Medical Oncology
The University of Texas MD Anderson Cancer Center
Houston, Texas

Kevin Madden, MD
Associate Professor of Palliative, Rehabilitation, and Integrative Medicine
The University of Texas MD Anderson Cancer Center
Houston, Texas

Laura Meyer, BA, MSW
PHD student in Health & Behavioral Sciences
University of Colorado, Denver
Denver, Colorado

Oluchi C. Oke, MD
Assistant Professor of General Medical Oncology
The University of Texas MD Anderson Cancer Center
Houston, Texas

Reverend Asa W. Roberts Jr., DEDMIN
Chaplain, Spiritual Care and Education
The University of Texas MD Anderson Cancer Center
Houston, Texas

Kimberson C. Tanco, MD
Associate Professor of Palliative, Rehabilitation, and Integrative Medicine
The University of Texas MD Anderson Cancer Center
Houston, Texas

Shiao-Pei Weathers, MD
Associate Professor of Neuro-Oncology
The University of Texas MD Anderson Cancer Center
Houston, Texas

Donna S. Zhukovsky, MD
Professor of Palliative, Rehabilitation, and Integrative Medicine
The University of Texas MD Anderson Cancer Center
Houston, Texas

Foreword

FROM A VERY early age, I learned about caring for patients through my dad, who was a cardiologist in Rosario, Argentina. On one hand, he was a lover of science and evidence-based medicine, but on the other hand he placed great importance on the many stories his patients shared about their travels, family issues, and what they did for fun. By hearing my dad recall these stories, I started learning that there was more to medicine than diseases. We would talk over dinner every day and over lunch on many days, and I could tell that he was more motivated to connect with his patients on a human level than he was to dwell on details of medical science, something that he was almost embarrassed to admit. He would visit the homes of his patients who were too ill to travel to his office, which was rarely done at that time. Sometimes he let me tag along, and I would wait in the car as he saw patients. We usually went to about three homes, after which he would take me on an excursion to do something fun that I wanted to do. Through this process, I began to understand that there were two sides to medicine: the evidence-based scientific side, which is what I later learned in medical school and residency, and the human side. Even as a young boy, I began to see the human impact of disease and the healing potential of doctors.

During medical school and residency, I did not pay a lot of attention to humanism, because I was too absorbed by the science of medicine. However, when I became an oncology fellow in Buenos Aires, my views changed. I had a sentinel case of a woman with ovarian cancer who had received treatment in her community and came to see us for more treatment options. She was frail and cachectic but nonetheless was always very warm and engaging, hugging us enthusiastically at the beginning and end of each visit. She never displayed even a hint of self-pity and instead seemed more nurturing toward us than we were toward her. The things I remember most about my meetings with her are my feelings of incompetence and guilt. We had so little to offer at that time to treat her cancer, which was the only way I could think of to relieve her suffering. I started to question how we were learning oncology and wondered why we didn't know how to better relieve suffering in ways other than shrinking tumors. One day she told us, "I have three school-aged children at home, and I want to see each of them get married and have children of their own. I can't die before I hold my grandchildren in my arms." I froze in silence, at a complete loss for words. I think I eventually mumbled something about trying more chemotherapy if she got stronger and gained weight.

During my oncology fellowship in Argentina, I started challenging a lot of my own beliefs and knowledge, and I started reading and studying about what we could do to help people who are suffering. It took me that long to really understand that there is a person behind every story who should be the focus of our attention, not just the tumor. I also learned very rapidly that nobody around me knew anything about the human aspects of medicine. Most of my mentors and peers at that time felt almost contemptuous of doctors who focused on the illness experience rather than the disease. They felt that discussion of such matters was unnecessary on rounds and had no bearing on clinical decision making. All the discussion on rounds was very formal and focused on scientific evidence. In fact, most people considered discussions about personhood as almost unprofessional.

I started wondering how I could learn more about the human side of things, and I was disappointed to find few options. I knew I would have to proactively seek opportunities to learn more. One day while seeing patients, I found out that a professor from Italy whom I had never heard of, Vittorio Ventafridda, was scheduled to give a lecture about palliative issues in Buenos Aires. Ventafridda was an anesthesiologist who was doing all kinds of nerve blocks for pain control. Then one day he had this revelation that treating pain purely as an electrical problem of nerve conduction made no sense, since there was a suffering person behind the pain. So he stopped doing procedures and focused more on treating people. Ventafridda's seminar was scheduled to be given at a large academic medical center in Buenos Aires. I desperately wanted to hear him speak, so I asked another oncology fellow in the program to cover my patients to allow me to take the bus downtown to the lecture hall. This was during winter, so it was freezing in this huge auditorium at the medical school. The venue could easily have accommodated several hundred people, but when I arrived, there were literally only four people at the venue. Even the people who had invited him did not care to show up. Ventafridda had traveled all the way from Milan to give a groundbreaking lecture, and there were only five people in this huge auditorium. I hadn't even paid registration to the Congress; I just snuck in. Despite the tiny audience, Ventafridda gave the most extraordinary and passionate talk, speaking the entire hour while barely pausing for breath. He discussed many things that finally resonated with me concerning the importance of personhood management. More importantly, he impressed upon me the power that one passionate person can have on an impressionable young mind. One never knows who might attend a seminar and really take advantage. There may be 1,000 people present or only five, but it only takes one energized person to carry the torch and move the field forward to inspire countless others.

And so, as an oncologist in training, I was initially touched by a loving patient with ovarian cancer who traveled all the way to Buenos Aires from her small town in the interior of Argentina with bright eyes and a heart full of hope. Then I was energized by a passionate physician from Italy who was forging new paths in pain management by focusing on people rather than on their diseases. I then decided that's what I wanted to do with my career.

It wasn't easy to embark on a career focused on personhood, because there were no role models, mentors, or programs in Argentina or anywhere else in South America. I had to apply for faculty positions in many places around the world, 52 institutions to be exact. After much rejection, I was finally contacted by Neil MacDonald, who was the director of the cancer center in Edmonton, Canada. Without knowing me, he replied to me in a letter to say he didn't do the kind of care I was proposing, but that he wanted to implement it in his cancer center. He suggested I work there for a year, open a clinic, and see what we could do. And that's exactly what happened. Neil and I learned together. I learned from him the importance of having somebody who has your back. It would have been impossible for me to accomplish anything meaningful if he had not protected me and created a nurturing environment. He was a true visionary who decided to take a chance. So, if a department head in medical oncology or radiation oncology wanted something from me, Neil told them, "Don't bother Eduardo. Just send him some patients and leave him alone to do his work." Then, Neil would take the flak for me and discuss whatever the colleague wanted, perhaps a new radiation therapy machine or a new chemotherapy program. Neil insulated me from all the noise and distraction and allowed me to focus on what I thought was very useful for our patients. We had to be very resourceful to build our program in palliative medicine, for instance by converting a decrepit old hospital ward into a clinic. I thought that would be the whole trajectory of my career and that I would grow old in Edmonton. Then, after working in Edmonton for 15 years, I received a call out of the blue from John Mendelson who told me, "I want to bring what you are doing in Edmonton to MD Anderson Cancer Center in Houston." At that time in the late 1990s, we still did not have a palliative specialty in the United States and there was no such thing as palliative fellowship. Basically, we did not have any of the things we have now other than a clear idea of where we wanted to go, which was to focus on patient-centered care. We wanted to emphasize the suffering experience rather than the disease.

I still often reminisce about the strong influence my dad had on me: the way I spoke with him at dinner time, and the way he told me stories of his patients and the things that mattered most to them. Although he wanted me to focus on medical science, I could see that he was more interested in humanity, which made an indelible impression on me. When he died rather suddenly at the age of 79, he was still seeing a few patients, so I was asked to clear out his office of diplomas, books, and other keepsakes. As I did, I discovered a most extraordinary thing that I did not know about him when he was alive. Over his many years of practice, he accumulated countless gifts brought by grateful patients, some of which were beautiful or even valuable, and others that were downright ugly. He kept most of these gifts in a closet in his office, since he did not have room to display all of them and had no inclination to display the more garish ones. And when he knew a patient was scheduled to come for an appointment, he would pull that patient's present out, no matter how tacky it was, and display it on his desk or on the wall to honor the patient and to give the impression that the gift was displayed permanently. And then, when the patient left, he would store it back in the closet. When I cleaned out his office, I found many of those objects, most of which were labeled with the patient's last name so he could keep track of them. He never discussed this practice with me or anyone else, but he must have understood that honoring his patients by displaying their gifts would have a healing effect. I keep an old black-and-white picture on my desk at work that shows my dad as a young physician presenting a paper at a conference. My time with my dad when I was in elementary school riding around with him in the car as he made house calls was formative for me. I never entered patients' houses back then, but later after I was able to drive, he would dispatch me to some of his patients' homes to do EKGs for him to read back in his office. This was a kind of weekend job for me and was also a way for me to get my first glimpse at people's lives in their homes. More importantly, I believe my home EKG visits were therapeutic for my dad's patients, because they felt as if a little part of their doctor, his son no less, cared enough to travel to see them.

Now, over 30 years into my career as a palliative specialist, I have learned many things about how to care for patients compassionately. The biomedical knowledge comes relatively easily: all I need to do is read the literature as much as I can every day. In contrast, my ability to speak with my patients and their families compassionately has come in a much more haphazard fashion, primarily by watching others in action, copying the phrases and strategies that seem to work best, and practicing in isolation through trial and error. This process has been fraught with mistakes and many awkward moments, but I eventually developed my own style that seems to work well and continues to evolve. I have also honed my relational skills by reading many books, chapters, and scholarly articles about breaking bad news and other communication challenges. However, none of those resources are nearly as engaging, relevant, or practical for busy clinicians as this book.

This book could not come at a better time. Most doctors do not feel as though they have permission or time to dwell in the emotional, psychosocial domain, and even those who do may lack the skills they need to do so effectively. Electronic medical records make matters even worse by functioning more as billing systems and repositories of lab data than as collections of important narrative about patients' humanity. If anything, electronic records dehumanize the patient narrative with smart phrases and templates and the like. Ideally, we should document something that gives insight into the patient's humanity, such as the type of guitar he most enjoys playing, or her plans for a religious pilgrimage, or his studies to become a banker. Then, we have something to talk about when they visit, like the gifts stacked up in my dad's office closet. In my view, clinicians are more aware of the need to be empathic than ever before, but barriers exist that prevent them from meeting that need. Back in the 1980s and 1990s, doctors did not even understand the importance of being empathetic, even though they had more time for their patients and therefore relatively more opportunity to honor their stories.

Now, doctors and other providers spend so much time typing and clicking that they have little time for imagining what the other person is feeling and responding to those emotions, which is the essence of empathy. What the medical world needs now more than anything is a very practical guide for clinicians to help them respond empathically under the most challenging circumstances and under the excruciating time pressure we all experience every day. Besides the conceptual grounding, empathic practice also requires an extensive repertoire of empathic phrases that promote connection between us and our patients during their most emotional and vulnerable moments. Most doctors lack such a repertoire. This book is like none other, since it engages readers with compelling stories that vividly illustrate the highly charged situations faced by patients and those who care for them. It then offers extensive dialogue with the actual words and phrases that promote empathy in clinical practice under real-life conditions, when time is limited, computers are present in every room, and stress levels are high. Everything written here brings best communication practices to life for busy clinicians. I wish I had this book when the frail woman with recurrent ovarian cancer traveled all the way to Buenos Aires and put her hope in me. If so, I would have known how to respond to her when she said, "I can't die before I hold my grandchildren in my arms."

Eduardo Bruera, MD, FAAHPM
Professor and Chair, Department of Palliative, Rehabilitation and Integrative Medicine and F.T. McGraw Chair in the Treatment of Cancer, Division of Cancer Medicine, The University of Texas MD Anderson Cancer Center, Houston, Texas

Preface

I REMEMBER SITTING in a large auditorium for an introductory biology course as a Stanford undergraduate in 1979 on the day when an esteemed member of the faculty named Paul Berg was scheduled to give the lecture. A black wooden captain's chair emblazoned with the Stanford logo awaited his arrival at center stage. Just as class was about to begin, I felt the unholy sensation of the earth moving in waves beneath me as a large chandelier swayed menacingly overhead. Not knowing what was happening, I nervously looked at my friend Bill in the seat next to me. Bill was raised in California, so he just shrugged and matter-of-factly said, "Earthquake," as I silently prayed for the chandelier above us to remain attached to the ceiling. A few moments later, Dr. Berg sat in that elegant chair as he described his lab group's success at cloning a gene for the first time, a discovery for which he shared the Nobel Prize in Chemistry in 1980. That minor earthquake paled in comparison to Dr. Berg's earth-shattering discovery, which ushered in the era of molecular genetics and created a tectonic shift in medical science. I quickly became enthralled by stories of scientific discovery and vowed to join the molecular genetic revolution. I spent 20 hours per week in a research lab during my final 2 years of college and experienced the thrill of discovery for the first time. My career trajectory was set: I would be a physician-scientist.

A Passion for Research

A few years later, I started medical school at Baylor College of Medicine in Houston, Texas. One day during our first year, I chatted with a few friends during a 10-minute break between lectures as we stood beneath a larger-than-life portrait of Michael E. DeBakey, MD, in the lobby of the building bearing his name. DeBakey was the great cardiovascular surgeon and medical statesman who was a major driving force behind the creation and growth of the school. As we chatted, one of our classmates, whose father was a cancer researcher at a neighboring institution, breathlessly ran up to us and declared, "My father just cured cancer." She had just learned that her father had contributed to the discovery of oncogenes, a monumental discovery that elucidated cancer's molecular underpinnings but hardly represented the cure that she imagined. Advances in cancer diagnosis and treatment have mostly been incremental rather than monumental over the ensuing 40 years. Regardless, the discovery of oncogenes further stirred my passion for a career in science, and finding a cure to cancer was the ultimate scientific prize.

After graduating from Baylor College of Medicine, I moved to the University of Texas Southwestern Medical School and Parkland Hospital for internal medicine residency. I was drawn to Parkland because of its reputation as a rigorous program where medical luminaries like Don Seldin seamlessly merged their basic research with patient care. At Southwestern, science was king. One day post-call as a second-year resident, my new attending for the month, Dr. Michael Brown, arrived near the nurses' station at 10 am to begin morning rounds. Dr. Brown and Dr. Joe Goldstein had just received the Nobel Prize in Physiology or Medicine two years before (1985) for their discoveries concerning the regulation of cholesterol metabolism. Science and medicine were so inextricably linked at Southwestern that even Nobel laureates took turns attending on the wards for at least a few weeks every year. One of the first patients the intern presented that morning was a man with a history of heavy alcohol consumption with cirrhosis who was admitted overnight with a GI bleed. At first glance, the man was just another GI bleeder with esophageal varices due to portal hypertension, so I expected Dr. Brown to wave off detailed discussion and quickly proceed to the next patient. Instead, he thought about the patient for a few seconds and asked, "Did Mr. Smith have Keiser Fleisher rings?" I stood in stunned silence as I reached back into the far recesses of my memory and recalled that Keiser Fleisher rings are the ophthalmic manifestation of Wilson's disease, a rare, inherited derangement of copper metabolism that causes cirrhosis. Dr. Brown was a brilliant scientist and an equally brilliant clinician who reaffirmed the glory of biomedical knowledge. Dr. Brown was the physician-scientist superstar I wanted to become one day.

The Siren Call of Humanism

While the allure of basic biomedical research energized me during the formative years of my career, the human side of medicine also began to whisper in my ear, almost as if humanity was competing with science for my love and affection. I remember discussing the case of an elderly woman with progressive refractory squamous cell cancer of the nasopharynx on rounds at Parkland one day. My attending that month was Leonard Madison, an endocrinologist who had a heart of gold and cared deeply about his mentees and even more deeply about his patients. My third-year resident was already accepted into one of the country's most prestigious oncology fellowship programs, so he enthusiastically listed the many chemotherapy regimens the woman had received and plans for additional treatment. As the entire team followed Dr. Madison into the woman's room, he walked directly to her bedside, reached for her hand, and leaned over, ignoring the overwhelming odor that arose from the gaping hole in the center of her face created by the cancer. He then gently stroked her hand and said, "Mrs. S, I'm Dr. Madison, and I am here with the medical team to see how you are. Is there anything we can do for you today?" The woman just lay there inanimately. After waiting a few seconds, he asked, "Ma'am, are you comfortable now?" She remained silent and still. He then asked, "Is there anyone you want to be here with you today? Any family?" When she again failed to respond, he patted her hand one final time and said, "Dear, we are here to help you anyway possible. Please let us know if you need anything." Once we were back in the hallway out of earshot, Dr. Madison turned to my resident and quietly said, "Please, just keep her comfortable." Our unofficial motto during residency at Parkland was "No one dies on my watch," but Dr. Madison urged us that day to focus on this woman's humanity and dignity rather than on chasing unrealistic dreams of cure. At that time, in 1986, I had never heard the word "palliative," but Dr. Madison illustrated its meaning and opened my eyes to the power of caring and humanism.

I continued to follow the siren call of science by completing a molecular genetics fellowship between Internal Medicine residency at Southwestern and Oncology fellowship at Johns Hopkins Oncology Center. When I arrived at Johns Hopkins in 1991, the oncology center was separated physically, administratively, and financially from the main hospital. As a result, we oncologists had no access to a dedicated intensive care unit. When one of our hospitalized patients became critically ill, as they often did, we rolled a ventilator into the room and functioned as de facto intensivists. This arrangement was not problematic for the fellows, since we had all just finished 3 years of internal medicine residency and were comfortable with routine aspects of critical care. We also knew when to call our critical care colleagues for help.

Awakening to the Importance of Goals of Care

For a while, I just did what I was trained to do: address laboratory abnormalities, adjust ventilator settings, review imaging studies, and prescribe supportive therapy in hopes that my patients would recover. However, over time, I began to see these critically ill patients as much greater than the sum of their many biomedical abnormalities. Even though nearly all of them were unconscious on ventilators, I saw them as people rather than just as patients, and I got to know them through the many pictures on their nightstands and windowsills and through their families' stories. I began to wonder whether our highly technical and reductionist approach was accomplishing anything meaningful. I anecdotally observed that essentially all patients with advanced cancer who required intensive care, especially those who required mechanical ventilation, died during the hospitalization or shortly after. I began to view death in an ICU and particularly on a ventilator as undignified and inhumane, at least for patients whose death seemed inevitable. I also perceived the experience to be traumatic for family members and for the healthcare team who were repeatedly exposed to it. I began to ask myself why our default approach was to offer all heroic measures rather than to allow natural death, even for patients whose long-term survival seemed impossible. As my interest in this topic grew, I began a retrospective study to determine the outcome of mechanical ventilation for patients with hematological malignancies and published the resulting manuscript with the help of collaborators. That was my "Sunday project," the one I worked on nights and weekends when I wasn't working in the research lab during the latter years of my oncology fellowship at Hopkins. Not surprisingly, we found that patients with refractory malignancy who needed mechanical ventilation had dismal outcomes, consistent with my clinical experience. While I waged the War on Cancer, the sound of humanity whispered ever more loudly in my ear.

Words Can Heal, and Words Can Harm

A few years later when I took my first faculty position at Baylor College of Medicine, my alma mater, I focused primarily on basic and translational research and ran my own federally funded lab for several years. Despite spending about 80% of my time in the lab, I attended on the oncology consult service a few months per year and on the internal medicine service one month per year just as faculty members at Parkland had. I distinctly remember an encounter on rounds that forever changed the way I approach conversations with patients. The medical oncology fellow and I were asked to see a middle-aged man with a history of colon cancer that was resected several months before and who was admitted for jaundice. CT revealed recurrent cancer in the form of several liver metastases, so we had the unenviable task of discussing CT results and recommending a course of treatment. The fellow, who was very bright and personable, led the conversation. It sounded something like this:

"Mr. Smith, we are from the oncology service, and we are here to discuss your CT results and treatment options. Your CT showed innumerable lesions in both lobes of your liver that represent recurrent cancer, which explains your jaundice. Your hyperbilirubinemia precludes treatment with the standard chemotherapy regimen, so we will have to adapt your treatment accordingly. I am sorry to say your cancer is not curable." Then without pausing to let this profound news sink in, he attempted to reassure the man by saying, *"but it is treatable."*

He then proceeded in similar fashion, using jargon to discuss imaging studies, bloodwork, and treatment options, including possible side effects of treatment. He finally handed the man a chemotherapy consent form to sign. He never asked the patient what he understood about his illness or whether he wanted a family member or someone else in his close inner circle to be part of the conversation, let alone allowed him to ask questions or express his fears, priorities, or hopes. As I watched the encounter, I realized it was going terribly wrong despite the young doctor's good intentions and pleasant demeanor. That moment was pivotal for me, the point when I decided to find out what it is about our conversations with patients that can be therapeutic, and conversely, what can be harmful. By that point in my career, the sounds of humanity that were once whispers in my ear had grown to exhortations.

Focus on Communication Skills Training

I then gradually phased out my lab research program and began to study the patient-clinician communication literature as voraciously as I had studied the basic science literature. I learned that most patients want realistic prognostic information to make well-informed decisions about their care, regardless of how upsetting that information is. Sensitive conversations should ideally occur incrementally over multiple meetings, preferably early in the disease trajectory and often in the presence of others in the patient's close inner circle. Many studies have shown that the most effective clinical conversations allow space for patients to pose technical questions, describe their priorities, and express negative emotions, including fear, sadness, grief, and helplessness. I now know that when clinicians respond to strong negative emotions with technical information or false reassurance rather than with empathy, they speak a language that is entirely unintelligible to the patient. Empathy is the universal language of emotion that allows us to connect meaningfully with our most vulnerable patients.

A short time later, I met Walter Baile, a psychiatrist and healthcare communication expert at MD Anderson Cancer Center, where I was recruited to join the faculty in General Oncology in 2008. Immediately after I arrived at MD Anderson, Walter suggested I participate in Oncotalk Teach, an NIH-funded program to teach oncology faculty how best to teach oncology fellows communication skills. Oncotalk Teach consisted of two 3-day retreats separated by 6 months during which faculty worked in small groups facilitated by one of the principal investigators, including Tony Back, Bob Arnold, Walter Baile, Kelly Fryer-Edwards, and James Tulsky. Oncotalk Teach was transformative for me. I considered myself a good communicator before attending, but I gained enormous insight regarding my communication and teaching skills from thoughtful feedback I received from my peers and small group facilitator, James Tulsky, a world-class clinician educator, researcher, and administrator. I now know that the best educators are much like coaches who begin by building a solid conceptual framework with learners, then model key skills in the right measure, create a safe environment in which to practice skills, observe learners in action, ask learners to reflect on the experience, offer objective feedback tailored specifically to the learner's needs, and establish future goals. This coaching paradigm was unlike any I had experienced before as a learner or as a teacher but has guided me since.

Career Evolution

The Department of General Oncology at MD Anderson Cancer Center proved to be fertile ground for my professional development, because it gave me the opportunity to work in a wide variety of clinical settings where I honed my own communication skills and my ability to teach them. I was medical director of the International Cancer Assessment Center where I cared for patients from many different cultures, spent about 20% of my time practicing integrative medicine, and devoted another 20% attending on the Center for Targeted Therapy (phase I) hospital service, where I discussed goals of care, code status, and end-of-life issues with nearly every patient. I also supervised medical oncology fellows one day per week in their continuity clinics, where I applied the Oncotalk Teach model.

Being at MD Anderson in the same academic building as Walter Baile was also a godsend. Walter and I collaborated on many educational initiatives at MD Anderson and elsewhere, the most notable of which were "Clinical Leadership Rounds" and "Difficult Conversations," recurring series of communication skills workshops for palliative medicine fellows and medical oncology fellows, respectively. We published a description of "Difficult Conversations" in *Academic Medicine* in 2014 and the process of integrating narrative into the curriculum in the *Journal of Cancer Education* in 2018. After a few years in general oncology, my career had evolved so completely from physician-scientist and cancer researcher to clinician-educator and humanist that I moved full time to the Department of Palliative, Rehabilitation, and Integrative Medicine at MD Anderson in 2012 and have remained there since.

The Power of Stories

A patient whom I saw in the International Cancer Assessment Center changed the course of my career dramatically. He was a middle-aged man from Kuwait with stage III rectal cancer whom I evaluated and then referred to Dr. Michael Overman, the gastrointestinal medical oncologist who coordinated his multidisciplinary care and administered his chemotherapy. The standard of care for this patient included preoperative radiation combined with chemotherapy, surgery, and postoperative combination chemotherapy for several months, a complex regimen that any patient would find difficult to understand. The great challenge for this man was that he was deaf, mute, and did not communicate with standard sign language, which made traditional informed consent impossible. Fortunately, he was highly intelligent and personable, so we were able to work closely with the patient's family, a language assistant, and a medical ethicist to develop a sound game plan that yielded an excellent outcome. The situation was so memorable for both of us that Dr. Overman suggested we collaborate to write a reflective essay describing it, which we published in the *Journal of Clinical Oncology* "Art of Oncology" section in 2011. Until then, neither of us had written a reflective piece, but after receiving positive feedback from many colleagues who read the essay, I quickly saw the potential of such stories to serve as enduring educational resources to teach communication skills, particularly empathy. I then published a few more such essays in the *Annals of Internal Medicine*, *Journal of Clinical Oncology*, and other journals and attended a multiday workshop at Columbia University Department of Narrative Medicine with Rita Charon and her outstanding group to learn more about the field. Since then, I have published several other reflective essays in the medical literature, often in collaboration with colleagues, and have integrated narrative into many of my communication skills seminars and workshops. One of the basic premises of this book is that stories engage learners and complement conceptual frameworks perfectly to help clinicians build communication skills.

Building a Repertoire of Empathic Language

Over the past several years while teaching communication skills, I have noticed that many clinicians respond to emotionally charged clinical conversations with biomedical, factual information or false reassurance rather than with empathy. The communication style displayed by the medical oncology fellow I observed on rounds at Baylor was hardly the exception. The literature confirms that clinicians, particularly physicians, miss many empathic opportunities, even though strong emotions permeate almost every conversation they have with patients. Clinicians understand on a conceptual level that empathy entails "standing in the other person's shoes" or imagining what another person is thinking or feeling, yet they still find it difficult to occupy the emotional space with patients. There are several possible explanations for this apparent lack of empathy. One is that many clinicians have been taught to remain emotionally distant from patients to maintain composure and objectivity. I remember a small group session I facilitated in our "Difficult Conversations" series a few years ago that included an oncology fellow with an impressive research pedigree. He was a few years older than the other fellows, having earned a PhD and done a research postdoc before returning to clinical training. He seemed stoic and reserved during our large group sessions. However, when he assumed the role of physician caring for a young woman dying of breast cancer in our small group role play, he suddenly became overwhelmed with emotion and started crying. I learned from that experience that some clinicians who appear to be the most detached and scientific on the surface are actually the most sensitive and caring inside. I also learned to be empathic rather than judgmental toward colleagues who struggle to realistically discuss prognosis and goals of care with their patients. Discussing code status and transitioning to a purely palliative strategy is heart-wrenching work for anyone.

Clinicians may also miss many empathic opportunities because they lack a sufficient repertoire of empathic phrases with which to dive deeply into emotional conversations. If they say anything empathic, they often run out of steam after saying a few stock phrases, like "I cannot imagine how difficult this must for you" or any statement beginning with "I wish." The NURSE acronym, a conceptual framework published by Pollak and colleagues in the *Journal of Clinical Oncology* in 2007, can be used as a teaching tool to address this challenge. The N in NURSE stands for naming the emotion, the U for understanding or validating the emotion, R for respect, S for support, and E for exploring emotions further to encourage more expression. The investigators characterized empathic responses in these categories as continuer statements that allow patients to continue expressing emotions and found that when oncologists respond with them, patients have less anxiety and depression and report greater satisfaction and adherence to therapy. I find that respectful empathic statements, symbolized by the R in NURSE, are particularly powerful for helping me connect with patients. Examples of such statements include "I respect your fighting spirit," "I respect your strong religious faith," and "I respect the love between you and your family." This book contains many more such examples. These are healing words as long as they are heartfelt. The challenge for many clinicians is to incorporate these and many more empathic expressions into their practice to occupy the emotional space with the patient for as long as the patient will let them. Empathic expression should be more than just "one and done."

I had an epiphany a couple of years ago that stimulated me to write this book. I was attending in the palliative care unit at MD Anderson, and as usual our team included two palliative medicine fellows and a medical oncology fellow who was completing his required palliative elective in our department, in addition to a pharmacist, counselor, chaplain, social worker, and nursing team. Alex Andreev, the medical oncology fellow, approached me one day after rounds and said, in essence, "I understand what empathy is, and I am impressed by how empathy helps you and others in your department connect with your patients, but I often cannot think of the right words to say when patients and families become emotional. Will you please give me a list of empathic phrases that I can memorize and use in my encounters?" When Dr. Andreev asked me for a list of phrases to memorize, I realized that such a list could be a precious resource for many clinicians, whose training involves memorizing huge quantities of factual information. Dr. Andreev is a physician-scientist who had the insight to know that clinicians can use their strong powers of memorization to strengthen their humanistic skills. He and I published a reflective essay in the *Journal of Clinical Oncology* "Art of Oncology" section in

2020 that describes our work together that month. The essay concludes as follows:

These observations, along with some profound patient encounters, led me to see that we have the potential to offer our patients a gift that is arguably as powerful and meaningful as targeted therapy or immunotherapy—the gift of humanity. If I can undergo this transformation, anyone can.

A short time later, Shine Chang PhD and Carrie Cameron PhD asked me to serve as an advisor for Laura Meyer, a college graduate who was accepted into their NCI-funded Cancer Prevention Research Training Program (CPRTP) Summer Internship. Laura has since completed her masters in social work and recently embarked on doctoral studies. Our goal for the summer was to develop a list of conversational challenges that often arise in the care of seriously ill patients and potential empathic responses to each challenge, as requested by Dr. Andreev a few months before. Laura and I first reviewed existing books and journal articles pertaining to empathy to determine that nothing like our proposed practical guide to empathic responding was already available. I then generated a list of scenarios and proposed empathic responses from my own practice as an oncologist and palliative doctor. We then built upon that foundation by anonymously surveying 44 palliative clinicians, including physician and non-physician providers at MD Anderson Cancer Center. We asked them to give examples of the conversations they find most challenging in their practice and then merged their responses with the original list as well as examples from the literature to create a more comprehensive list. We then assembled a focus group of five physicians, two advanced care providers, and one psychologist from the Department of Palliative Medicine at MD Anderson Cancer Center to get feedback about the format, themes, scenarios, and suggested empathic responses in the draft guide. Scenarios fell into several thematic categories, including denial, prognosis, existential concerns, difficult family dynamics, impact of illness on family, and nonmedical opiate use. We then formatted the list as a prototype for a clinician's pocket guide and approached Karen Edmonson, who at the time was a content editor for McGraw Hill, to gauge interest in the project. Karen and her colleagues were enthusiastic, but they requested that we write a full book rather than just a pocket guide. Other editors at McGraw Hill subsequently worked with us on this project.

My next challenge was to decide how to convert a very practical list of empathic phrases for clinicians into a full manuscript. I knew I did not want this book to be another philosophical, theoretical, or technical look at clinical empathy, but rather an engaging, real-life resource for busy clinicians. I decided that the same narrative approach that I had used to write reflective pieces for the *Journal of Clinical Oncology* and other journals was best suited to the task. I also decided that I wanted this book to reflect the viewpoints of a culturally diverse group of clinicians from a variety of medical disciplines rather than just my viewpoints or the views of palliative clinicians. The authors include five medical oncologists, six palliative physicians, a surgical oncologist, a chaplain, a social worker, an infectious disease physician, a pediatrician, a clinical psychologist, and an ophthalmologist. Many of the first authors were born and raised in other countries, including Canada, Germany, Ghana, Guatemala, Nigeria, Pakistan, the Philippines, and Taiwan. The authors represent nearly an equal mix of men and women who are at various stages of career development. Each chapter is anchored by a true but anonymized story that describes a challenging clinical scenario from the first author's clinical practice and relevant personal details about each author that helped shape their approach to empathic practice. This book ends with the concise pocket guide to empathic expression, the seed from which this book grew. I hope you will find this collection of real stories inspirational and enlightening.

Daniel E. Epner

Acknowledgments

I AM INDEBTED to Karen Edmondson for seeing the potential in this project from day one and for enthusiastically guiding me through its early stages of development. Karen models the same empathy that I hope to foster in clinicians who read this book. Many thanks to the editorial staff at McGraw Hill for skillfully helping me carry this book across the finish line.

Eduardo Bruera is a constant source of inspiration for his courage in blazing new trails in medical practice, for always focusing on person-centered care, and for making countless, high-impact contributions to the field of palliative medicine. Dr. Bruera has unfailingly promoted palliative care for the betterment of countless patients and their families. He is the most supportive, brilliant, passionate, and warm-hearted leader with whom I have ever worked. He also skillfully uses humor to lighten the mood under stressful circumstances, which arise every day in our care of seriously ill patients. I am deeply indebted to Dr. Bruera for enthusiastically supporting this project from start to finish.

My colleagues in the Department of Palliative, Rehabilitation, and Integrative Medicine at MD Anderson Cancer Center, including physicians, advanced practice providers, nurses, members of the psychosocial team, and the administrative team, have treated me and each other with the same respect and compassion as they treat our patients and colleagues in other departments. Working on the same team with them is extremely gratifying, because I know we practice medicine every day the way it should be practiced, namely by focusing on people's humanity rather than on their diseases.

I am also deeply indebted to the countless thousands of patients for whom I have cared over my long career. They inspire me with their courage in the face of terrifying circumstances, endlessly fascinating stories, and love for their families, friends, and spiritual communities. I have always been passionate about medical research and education, but my patients are what bring true meaning to my work.

Finally, my wife, Linda Epner, has been a constant guiding light who has nourished my body and soul for nearly four decades. She not only contributed a beautiful story to the current collection, but also generously gave her time in offering thoughtful and constructive feedback about several aspects of the book. She teaches me and our daughters, Margeaux and Eden, every day about compassion by generously sharing stories from her own ophthalmology practice in a community safety net clinic. Linda, Margeaux, and Eden are my constant sources of light and inspiration.

Introduction

EVERY PATIENT HAS an important story to tell. Rita Charon, in her landmark *New England Journal of Medicine* paper published in 2004, defined narrative competence as the ability to absorb, interpret, and respond to stories. This competence enables providers to practice with empathy, reflection, professionalism, and trustworthiness. Meaning is derived collaboratively, by the teller and listener, reader and writer, observer and observed, patient and physician. When a patient and clinician share a story, they experience it and derive meaning from it in their own ways. Each story becomes part of their lived experience and refines their worldview. Clinicians also have powerful stories to tell about their work, their families, mentors, hopes, dreams, and fears. This book sheds light on the interface between clinicians' stories and the stories of their patients.

As I considered how to structure this book, I initially envisioned asking contributors to focus on specific conversational challenges that commonly arise in their care of seriously ill patients. However, I soon realized that such a prescriptive approach would inhibit contributors from sharing the stories that are most meaningful to them and potentially most interesting and educational for readers. I therefore decided to take a more open approach by eliciting stories in much the same way as I elicit medical and psychosocial histories from patients. I gathered raw material for each chapter by interviewing each prospective contributor, asking them to "Tell me about a memorable encounter from your clinical work that illustrates your empathic practice." I allowed them to share their own stories, interrupting only rarely with the occasional brief question or comment to clarify and expand key points. My only other predetermined interview prompt was "Are there one or more people in your life, perhaps a family member, mentor, or colleague, who have informed your approach to empathic practice?" I then distilled the resulting raw transcripts from interviews into conceptual blocks, discarded extra material that did not propel the story forward, and assembled the resulting blocks into story structures that I thought would engage and inform busy clinicians. All stories were anonymized to protect the privacy of patients, families, and all clinicians other than the lead author and mentors whom they honor. Stories contain no personal health information or identifying data. All names used to refer to patients or their family members are not their real names. I remained true to each contributor's voice by including as much of their original language from interview transcripts as possible and incorporating their suggested modifications in final versions. The resulting collection of stories therefore represents the authentic voices of clinicians from a wide variety of cultural backgrounds and clinical disciplines and applies to a broad audience of clinicians at all stages of career development, from student to seasoned veteran.

The stories in this collection depict many common challenges, such as when patients and families harbor unrealistic prognostic expectations and are therefore considered to be "in denial" or when patients display nonmedical opiate use. However, not all chapters focus on challenging scenarios. Instead, some chapters focus primarily on how clinicians connect with patients by weaving empathy into the fabric of every encounter, not just difficult ones. Although this book offers readers extensive examples of empathic words and phrases with which to respond to emotional encounters, as intended, some chapters describe how actions can often be more empathic than even the most empathic words. Some stories describe the challenges that arise when clinicians face serious illness themselves or get stuck between the roles of clinician and family member as they care for an ill relative. Two chapters focus primarily on the role of spirituality and religion in enhancing empathic practice and addressing existential concerns. One story touches on a question commonly posed by patients' families, "What would you do if he were your father (or mother or other family member)?" A few chapters focus primarily on the unique challenges that arise when clinicians care for sick children or children of sick parents. Several stories highlight the outsize influence of mentors, parents, and grandparents on shaping clinicians' careers and development of their craft. Two chapters touch to varying degrees on the role of pets and other animals in strengthening connection between patients and their providers. Several chapters describe strategies for maintaining composure under duress, for instance when clinicians care for patients from chaotic or dysfunctional families or for those who suffer from mental illness. One story depicts a patient who remained distrustful of her medical team despite the fact that they went to great lengths to build trust, and the importance of focusing on process rather than on outcomes when defining success. I started writing this book at the beginning of the COVID-19 pandemic, so the pandemic is mentioned in almost every story. First and foremost, this book presents timeless stories from busy clinicians who face real-world challenges.

Besides compelling stories, this book also includes extensive practice points at the end of each chapter to solidify key teaching points. I included a brief clinician's guide to empathic expression as the last chapter to offer yet more examples of empathic language for addressing common clinical challenges, a few of which were not included in other chapters. This book can be read all in one sitting or one chapter at a time in any order, since each chapter stands on its own. Readers should learn from this book in the manner they see fit. The lessons presented here are timeless.

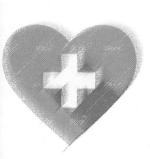

EMPATHY: REAL STORIES TO INSPIRE AND ENLIGHTEN BUSY CLINICIANS

1 Logic Only Takes You So Far: The Power of Emotional Connection

Faye M. Johnson and Daniel E. Epner

Blood and Chaos in the ICU

One patient I cared for about five or six years ago is indelibly seared in my brain. He was a man in his 40s with progressive refractory oral cavity cancer who had traveled from a foreign country to MD Anderson accompanied by his two brothers after receiving several types of salvage chemotherapy at other cancer centers and was desperately seeking additional treatment options. Before seeing the man, I reviewed his medical record and learned that my colleague, who was his primary outpatient oncologist at MD Anderson, had already discussed goals of care and prognosis and had recommended against additional cancer treatment, instead recommending a purely palliative approach. However, my colleague qualified his recommendation by saying that the patient could receive additional chemotherapy if his performance status remained good. The man and his brothers therefore insisted on more chemotherapy, which, unfortunately, caused his platelet count to drop precipitously and led to uncontrolled bleeding from his tumor, which was the reason he entered the hospital. The bleeding was due to diffuse tumor oozing and was therefore not amenable to cauterization or embolization. I was taking my turn covering the inpatient service for a few weeks, so I served as his attending physician during his hospitalization, responsible for overseeing all aspects of his care. I found this situation to be even more daunting than usual because I was meeting him for the first time in the hospital rather than having had the opportunity to establish rapport in the clinic. The patient and his brothers would have to decide within moments whether they trusted me with his life.

I have vivid memories of the scene at his bedside in the intensive care unit (ICU), where intensivists monitored him for uncontrolled bleeding and airway compromise due to the tumor. He and his brothers spoke no English, so I arranged for a language assistant to meet us outside the room. The ICU team was preparing to intubate him to protect his airway, and I had the task of discussing goals of care with an acutely unstable patient whom I had never met; who spoke no English; and who, due to the acute medical issues, could not have communicated even if he spoke English. I entered his room as soon as I arrived without engaging in the usual pleasantries with the language assistant and ICU team in light of the urgency of the situation. My eyes went immediately to the patient, who was struggling to breathe, choking on his own blood, and agitated. His face was a picture of sheer terror as he thrashed around the bed in a futile attempt to find a position in which he could breathe more comfortably. Every few seconds he coughed forcibly, spraying bright red blood in all directions. When one thinks about the "horrors of cancer," this scene is what may come to mind. I was desperate to find a way to help him avoid the final indignity and inhumanity of spending his last few days on a ventilator, but I had at most a few minutes to guide his brothers through this momentous decision. We either needed to intubate him quickly or allow him to die naturally.

I turned to his brothers, introduced myself, and described my role, at which point his brothers looked quizzically at each other, seemingly not understanding why I was speaking to them in a language they could not comprehend. The language assistant repeated my words, but his brothers ignored me and shouted the same phrase repeatedly, which I learned meant "Stop the bleeding! Stop the bleeding!" I concluded based on this brief interchange that he would almost certainly end up on a ventilator despite my efforts. I nonetheless did what I always do during a first meeting; I asked what they understood of their brother's condition, silently hoping they would express a clear understanding and a desire to focus purely on his comfort and dignity. Unfortunately, my hope was not answered because the older brother, who did most of the talking, turned to the language assistant and replied, "He has chemotherapy scheduled for next Tuesday. Can we give it to him now to stop his bleeding?" After a while, I reflexively started to speak to the language assistant directly because the brothers were ignoring me anyway. "Tell them that the chemotherapy actually caused his bleeding by lowering his platelet count and that we need to stop treating the tumor and discuss goals of care." The brothers considered this information for a moment and then asked, "How will we cure his cancer if we stop the chemotherapy?" Their question confirmed that I was not getting through to them despite my colleague's earlier efforts to communicate realistic goals of care. Either we were not doing a very good job of helping the patient and his brothers understand his grave prognosis during conversations in clinic or they were "in denial."

This conversation sticks in my mind because it was a very obvious and graphic example of how treating cancer beyond a certain point can actually hurt a person. Yet, despite the bloodbath occurring before our eyes, the brothers still insisted that the patient receive more treatment for his cancer. This was not some hypothetical bad thing. On one level, I understood that his brothers loved him and wanted the best for him, but the other part of my brain was silently screaming, "What on Earth are they thinking? This is barbaric! They are behaving so illogically." I took a deep breath to compose myself and responded to their request for more chemotherapy. "Unfortunately, we cannot cure your brother's cancer. Chemotherapy will only harm him." The language assistant hesitated for a moment to decide how best to express my very direct message and then uttered what seemed like at least five or six sentences in an apparent attempt to soften the blow. The brothers contemplated the language assistant's words and then replied, "God willing, he will make a full recovery. We are putting our faith in God." I had apparently made no progress in helping them understand that giving more chemotherapy would only hurt him. In addition, I was resigned to the fact that he would die on a ventilator. After several more minutes of watching the patient thrash about, gasp for air, and bleed profusely, the ICU team intubated him. As expected, he died two days later as his brothers, the ICU team, and I looked on helplessly. Those images will haunt me forever. This case, more than any other, taught me that even when the evidence is right in front of people, sometimes they still cannot comprehend it or, perhaps, refuse to understand. I find it incredibly frustrating when people will not see logic.

A Happier Ending

I also remember another patient and family whose approach to treatment contrasted sharply with that of the man and his brothers from a foreign country. He was a man in his 70s who was also from a foreign country and spoke no English who saw me in clinic to care for his very advanced oral cancer. Like the other man, his tumor had progressed despite several types of treatment and was now so advanced that it was almost surely incurable unless he experienced an unusually favorable response to treatment. Then, the full staging evaluation incidentally revealed a separate hepato-cellular carcinoma that was also probably incurable. The situation looked bleak, so I had a frank discussion with him and his adult son to explain that we can try chemotherapy and possibly later offer curative surgery for both cancers if he experienced a mirac-ulous response but that realistically, his odds of success were van-ishingly low. Armed with this warning, he nonetheless decided to take one cycle of chemotherapy to see how he would fare. He experienced such severe side effects that he ended up in the hos-pital for a month and nearly died. To make matters worse, neither of his tumors responded to treatment. When he finally recovered enough to return to my clinic a few weeks after discharge, he was very frail and was sedentary essentially all day. I reviewed his scans and lab data and summoned the courage to tell him that I did not think he was strong enough to receive more treatment, expecting him and his son to protest vehemently. Much to my relief, his son looked at me quizzically and asked, "What would be the point of putting him through that again?" I thought, "Finally, a patient and family who can see the logic of stopping chemotherapy." I wanted to kiss them for this insight. Granted, his outcome was not a suc-cess story from the oncological standpoint because his cancer pro-gressed and we could not do much about it. Nonetheless, he was able to enjoy his remaining days at home surrounded by loved ones rather than in an ICU. I think we were able to see eye-to-eye because they processed the facts I had presented to them logically and then decided to focus exclusively on quality of life.

The Power of Logic

I knew I wanted to be a doctor from a very young age. When I was in fourth grade, I described my career aspirations for a writing assignment:

> When I grow up I am going to medical school and learn how to be a doctor. I would be a pediatrician (a kid's

doctor). I would give children checkups. I wouldn't perform operations. I would have a big office with many rooms, a lobby for people to wait in with magazines, books and some toys. In the patient rooms we would have a bed and a piece of candy for all my patients.

When I started college, my dream of becoming a pediatrician was still alive. I envisioned spending long days in a clinic listening for congenital heart malformations in newborns, examining healthy toddlers while distracting them with stuffed animals, treating common infections, and offering wellness tips to adolescents. At that time, I focused entirely on becoming a clinician and initially had no interest in research. Nonetheless, like most premedical students, I worked in a lab as a practical strategy to buff up my medical school application. However, my entire outlook changed dramatically as soon as I entered the lab. I quickly found that creating new knowledge, no matter how incremental, energized me. I also loved designing my own experiments and then using logic to interpret the data. Molecular biology is like a big puzzle that one can logically assemble into a clear picture from the scattered pieces of raw data. As a physician scientist, I am very data-driven, so I nearly always use data to help my patients make well-informed decisions about treatment options. I often tell people that randomized controlled trials for lung cancer and many other cancers show that chemotherapy does more harm than good, shortens the life span, and erodes the quality of life for patients with poor functional status. Sometimes I come right out and tell patients with a poor performance status that the cancer is making them weak, so I seriously doubt that they will get stronger even if they recuperate for a few weeks.

Many people understand right away when I explain that their cancer is incurable. In fact, some even overreact and ask, "Why should I receive treatment and experience side effects if my cancer is incurable? I would rather go home and go fishing."

Then I have to say, "Hold on, let's try something because many people respond well and do not experience many side effects. You are not obligated to do many cycles of treatment if you tolerate the first one or two poorly. We can stop anytime you want." The cases when patients or family members are overzealous about treatment are often the most stressful, but I ironically find myself encouraging people who are hesitant to receive treatment to try it because I would readily recommend against treatment if I thought it was more likely to harm than help them. Most of them follow my advice and try treatment.

The Limits of Logic

I clearly remember a challenging discussion that suddenly changed my outlook about guiding patients in their clinical decision-making. The husband of a woman in the ICU with progressive mesothelioma repeatedly urged me to "do everything" even though she was clearly near death. We had to call ethics to intervene so the husband did not pressure us to do things that would increase the woman's suffering. He asked, "Why would anyone choose to stop treating the cancer?" At first, his question disarmed me because I thought anyone would understand what is arguably the most basic premise of medical practice, namely that all treatments pose potential risks. In this case, we risked depriving the patient of what little was left of her dignity and comfort. Then I quickly realized his question was not rhetorical. He had no medical background and therefore had no way of understanding the mysterious inner workings of the human body. He probably truly believed his wife could recover, even if recovery was all but impossible. The patient's husband asked, in essence, "What have we got to lose? She is dying anyway. We might as well go down fighting." Unfortunately, I had personally faced a similar situation, and I reflexively replied, "Well, you know, my dad chose to focus only on quality of life at the end of his life."

As soon as I uttered those words, an image of my father in his final days of life flashed before me. My father and mother divorced acrimoniously when I was young, so I had a complicated relationship with my father. I am in close contact with my mother, who lives only a few miles from my family and me, but my mom and my dad did not keep in touch. When my dad became frail and dependent at the end of his life, I was the only one around to care for him. He spent most of his retirement about a three hours' drive away, but I moved him into an apartment near our house when he was in his late 80s after he developed dementia and lung problems and got to the point where he was dwindling. The last time he went to the hospital, he was miserable. Every day when I visited his hospital room, he asked, "When can I go home?" Hearing him ask that question repeatedly broke my heart. After he was finally discharged, I asked him if he wanted to go back to the hospital if an urgent medical issue arose again in the future, and he said, "I hate being in the hospital. I never want to go back there." His dementia was mild so he was of sound mind when he made that decision. I explained that he could still get medications to maintain his quality of life if he stayed home, even if his life span was slightly shorter, and he agreed. My dad died peacefully about four years ago.

When I recall my conversation with the husband of the woman dying of mesothelioma in the ICU, I cannot say why I suddenly mentioned my father. Perhaps it was to "prove" to the husband that real people do indeed make decisions to not pursue aggressive care in favor of quality of life. However, I distinctly remember feeling an overwhelming urge to cry at that moment as I recalled the complicated relationship I had with my father after my parents' divorce so many years ago. Perhaps I was sad about all the missed opportunities, the many times my dad should have told me he loved me but did not, and the cold loneliness that separated us. I felt as though the sadness that I shackled in my heart so long ago suddenly broke free and tried to escape as tears. Crying would have been a healthy response at that moment, but I fought back the tears as I always do and continued the conversation. Fortunately, the patient's husband agreed to pivot toward a comfort strategy and forego more cancer treatment. That conversation helped me realize that strong emotions rather than logic guide people under the direst circumstances, almost as if emotions shove logic back into its neat, orderly home in the cerebral cortex and say, "Logic, you did your job. Now let me do mine." The patient's husband may have maintained a glimmer of hope that more chemotherapy would have actually helped his wife, but more than anything, he was grieving her impending death. Sadness, grief, and fear drove his decision rather than logic in the same way that my comment to him about my father originated from my heart rather than from my brain.

A New Perspective

Now I realize that logic and data, as powerful as they are, only get me so far, whether in my relationships with my patients and their families or in my laboratory research. Yes, I use my powers of analysis every day when I interpret laboratory data or make clinical decisions. However, truly novel scientific discoveries, whether profound or incremental, are born of intangibles, like inspiration and enlightenment. Who can explain how the process of pondering laboratory data stimulates the release of neurotransmitters within elaborate neural networks, which respond by reshaping and adapting, ultimately giving birth to novel ideas? The spark of discovery is as mysterious, powerful, and intangible as our emotional connections with our patients.

I also now realize that legacy does not depend upon longevity. My research accomplishments will certainly be an important part of my legacy because I ultimately do research for the betterment of humanity. I feel tremendous pride knowing that I am part of a grand network of countless scientists who have collaborated over many years to create meaningful clinical advances.

However, my impact on my children is arguably more important to my legacy than my work as a physician scientist. My children may not remember the scientific papers I publish, but I am sure they will always be proud of the example I set through my good deeds, my hard work, and my love for them. My legacy is safe whether I live just one more day or until the age of 100. Patients also have the freedom to create their own legacies, even if illness cuts their lives short, but we sometimes have to help them take stock of those legacies.

Lessons Learned

My approach to empathic practice continues to evolve as I gain clinical and life experiences and the perspective that grows from them. Every patient I see teaches me something about medicine, about humanity, and about myself. Now that I have experienced the normal worries, trials, and tribulations of family life, I can better imagine what my patients are going through, although I can never fully understand. Just imagining their experiences, such as the prospect of losing a loved one to cancer, is the essence of empathy. I like to think that I am wiser now than I was yesterday, last year, or 10 years ago.

For instance, when I think back to the international patient who bled to death from his oral cancer in the ICU, my perspective is different now that I have had kids, helped care for my dad at the end of his life, and cared for so many patients who faced the challenges of serious illness. I think now that if I saw that patient again, I would handle the situation differently. I would spend little or no time arguing medical details and focus more on empathizing with his family and respecting the fact that they loved him enough to bring him to the United States for care, which was a huge sacrifice. I would recognize that their hearts were in the right place and spend less energy feeling frustrated with their decisions. Finally, I would recognize that people who are scared and vulnerable are not necessarily "difficult," although a few probably are. Instead, they are trying to make the best decisions they can under nearly impossible circumstances.

How I Would Handle the Conversation If I Could Do It Again

The first thing I would do is close my eyes for just a few seconds to compose myself and remember that I am a well-trained, knowledgeable, skilled, and compassionate clinician, but I am only human. I can only do my best. I would then meet with the language assistant outside the room without the brothers present, either virtually, if the pandemic persists, or preferably in person, if circumstances permit. I would coordinate with the language assistant by explaining, "We are about to engage in a very emotional and difficult conversation during which we will discuss life and death matters. From what I can tell, this patient is near the end of his life. I will speak to the patient and his brothers with the utmost sensitivity, but I have to tell them the truth in order for them to make the best medical decisions. Please trust that I will speak the truth with compassion. You may feel the urge to soften the blow of what I say, but please translate my words as accurately as possible and add as little as possible."

I would then enter the room and begin by briefly introducing myself and my role to the patient's brothers, speaking to them directly throughout the conversation rather than in the third person through the language assistant, regardless of how they respond to me. I would then try to engage the brothers by encouraging them to express themselves, respond primarily with empathy rather than with medical facts and logic, and avoid the temptation to debate. Here is how it might sound:

"What do you want most for your brother at this point?"
Older brother: "We want him to be cured, of course."

"Yes, we all wish for cure, but I am concerned cure is not possible. I wish we had better options."

"We traveled 10,000 miles to your institution because you advertise that you can cure cancer, yet my brother is worse now than when he arrived. Look, he is bleeding to death. How will we stop the bleeding and cure his cancer?"

"I wish we could do more for him. I deeply respect how hard you have worked to care for your brother. I can tell how much you love him."

I can imagine his brother would continue as follows after a period of reflection and silence:

"We still pray for a miracle. His fate is up to God. We will never give up. We will fight for him no matter what."

"I respect your fighting spirit and your strong faith. Faith and hope are powerful medicines. What are you fighting for at this point?"

"I just said, we are fighting to cure my brother and take him back home to his wife and young children with his health completely restored."

"What else are you fighting for if we cannot achieve cure?"

"I want him to get strong enough to make it back home to see his family."

"That too is a beautiful dream. What do you want for him if he does not make it back home?"

I can imagine the brothers would be shocked by the thought of the patient dying far from home, so they would probably cry. I would wait silently to allow space for them to cry and wait for them to resume the conversation, even if it took a few minutes.

"What do we do now?"

"I think we need to focus on his comfort and dignity. His time is short."

"How short?"

"I cannot say for sure, but he could die at any moment, or he may live for a few days. That is my best guess."

"Days?!"

"I know that news must be shocking to you. I wish I had better news, but I think you need the truth, as hard as it is."

I would allow that profound news to sink in, and then continue:

"Most people who have cancer that is not responding to treatment decide to die naturally without machines and artificial support when their time comes. Did your brother ever share his wishes about this topic?"

"No."

"What do you think he would want?"

"I do not think he would want to be on a machine. There is no point to that."

"OK, we will do everything we can to fight for his comfort and dignity and support you and your brother the best we can. I can only imagine how hard this ordeal must be for you. You have both done an amazing job of supporting him. You have displayed tremendous strength and composure and should be proud of all you have done for him and the example you set for your family."

Then I would step out of the room, find a quiet place to gather my thoughts for a few moments, and tell myself what I always wished my father had told me before he died: "Faye, you did a great job in there. No one could have done better. Some problems are unsolvable. You used all your skills, knowledge, and compassion to help that man in the ICU and his brothers the best you could. By the way, my divorce from your mother was not your fault. I am sorry for the heartache I put you through.

I love you." Then, before moving on to the next patient, I would have allowed myself to cry, just a little.

PRACTICE POINTS

Key Reflections

- Gravely ill patients and their families are sometimes "illogical" when they make healthcare decisions, especially under dire circumstances.

- "Illogical" decisions are born of strong negative emotions, including fear, grief, anger, frustration, and sadness.

- Logical thought only goes so far in research and clinical medicine. Novel discoveries are born of inspiration, creativity, and enlightenment, just as great patient care is born of empathy, humanity, and compassion.

- Clinicians who use empathy in addition to logical discussion of biomedical facts are most likely to help patients and their families navigate the most emotionally charged decisions.

- Telling a patient who has no realistic chance of recovery, "We can offer more cancer treatment if you get stronger," creates false hope and is therefore deleterious.

Empathic Actions

- Physician scientists endure many years of hard work and discipline to acquire the extraordinary knowledge, skills, and insight needed to make novel discoveries for the betterment of their patients and humanity.

- Patient care is not for the faint of heart. Clinicians expose themselves to significant psychological and emotional trauma each day as they care for seriously ill patients, especially those who are approaching the end of life with a high symptom burden.

- Remaining present for patients when they experience the highest levels of distress and never abandoning them is arguably the most empathic action of any great clinician.

- Communicating the truth to patients and their families to facilitate informed decision-making is one of the basic tenets of ethical practice. Great clinicians share the truth sensitively and compassionately.

- Crying in small measure or otherwise showing authentic emotion is a healthy impulse for clinicians who care for seriously ill, vulnerable patients. Displaying authentic emotion is one way of revealing our humanity and compassion.

- Well-trained, knowledgeable, skilled, and compassionate clinicians should regularly remind themselves and their colleagues that they are only human. They cannot solve every problem. They can only do their best.

Empathic Expression

- "Yes, we all wish for cure, but I am concerned cure is not possible. I wish we had better options."

- "I wish we could do more for him. I deeply respect how hard you have worked to care for your brother. I can tell how much you love him."

- "I respect your fighting spirit and your strong faith. Faith and hope are powerful medicines. What are you fighting for at this point?"

- "What do you want most for your brother at this point?"

- "I think we need to focus on his comfort and dignity. His time is short."

- "I know that news must be shocking to you. I wish I had better news, but I think you need the truth, as hard as it is."

- "Most people who have cancer that is not responding to treatment decide to die naturally without machines and artificial support when their time comes. Did your brother ever share his wishes about this topic?"

- "We will do everything we can to fight for his comfort and dignity and support you and your brother the best we can."

- "I can only imagine how hard this ordeal must be for you."

- "You have both done an amazing job of supporting him. You have displayed tremendous strength and composure and should be proud of all you have done for him and the example you set for your family."

CHAPTER

2 | Code Blue

Sujin Ann-Yi and Daniel E. Epner

Dr. Ann-Yi is a licensed psychologist and marriage and family therapist in the Department of Palliative Medicine at MD Anderson Cancer Center with a background in family therapy and pediatrics. She spends most of her time as a consultant for hospitalized patients and works primarily with adults diagnosed with cancer with young children.

My pager almost never goes off, since colleagues in psychiatry handle psychiatric emergencies, such as suicidal or acutely agitated patients. So, when I received four pages in quick succession recently, I first thought they were wayward pages intended for psychiatry. When I dialed the first of the four numbers, someone on the oncology unit answered on the first ring: "Please come now ... patient died ... young daughter ... no family ... Spanish speaking." She was so distressed that she barely paused for breath, much like each of the other three callers, all of whom worked on the same unit. All four pages were clearly intended for me. Rather than try to piece together fragments of the story over the phone, I immediately went to the unit to assess the situation firsthand, climbing five flights of stairs to avoid waiting for an elevator. As I emerged from the stairwell, the scene in the hallway looked like a code blue. Clinicians in scrubs of various colors frenetically shuttled in and out of a room by the nurses' station as a chaplain huddled in the hallway with a few other clinicians, clerks, and administrators. A woman wearing black scrubs and a white coat, signifying her role as nurse manager, looked up from the mayhem, spotted me, and asked, "Dr. Ann-Yi?" Before I could answer, she directed me to a relatively quiet spot a few paces down the hallway to debrief me.

The patient was a young woman with progressive malignancy who was admitted through the emergency center for seizures related to newly discovered brain metastases. She had fought her illness bravely over several months, but her condition had declined so precipitously in recent days that she was no longer a candidate for more cancer treatment. It became clear to her oncologists and to everyone else caring for her that she was rapidly approaching death. She was initially alone in the hospital due to visitor restrictions related to the pandemic, but her care team allowed a compassionate exception for her four-year-old daughter and two family friends who had taken care of her during the hospitalization to come to the hospital for a visit. Shortly after her daughter arrived, the patient had a grand mal seizure and was postictal for a few minutes. She then awakened just long enough to tell her daughter, "I love you"; closed her eyes; and took her last breath.

Everyone knew the woman was gravely ill, but nobody thought she would die that suddenly. Of course, the little girl had no idea what had just happened because at her age, she did not understand the permanence of death. The patient's friends cried in the corner while averting their gaze from the body, paralyzed with indecision. Should they hug the little girl? What should they tell her? After a few seconds, one of the women left the room to tell someone in broken English what had happened. Not understanding the friend's words but nonetheless seeing panic in her eyes, the bedside nurse ran to assess the situation, found the patient unresponsive with no vital signs, and hustled back out to report the event up the chain of command, thus setting off the frenetic scene that I observed when I exited the stairwell.

After the initial shock of witnessing the deathbed scene, nurses and the attending doctor huddled to consider their next moves. The nurses knew the standard procedure for handling a death, but no one knew what to do with the patient's daughter, who had no relationship with her biological father and had no family available in the United States. Everyone assumed the patient's sister would take the child back to their home country, but she was still in transit and out of touch until her plane landed later that day. Suddenly someone recalled that the palliative/supportive care service has a psychologist who deals with such matters, at which point they frantically paged me.

I have counseled many thousands of patients and families under the direst circumstances, yet I almost always feel confident and prepared when I enter a room. When faced with sensitive situations like this, I usually speak with family members well ahead of time to learn who will continue to care for the child after a parent dies and what has already been communicated in addition to thoroughly reviewing the chart to learn a great deal about the patient's psychosocial history. In this crisis, however, I had no time to prepare, and I was terrified. I knew only the child's name and age and rudiments of her mother's medical history, so I had to assess on the fly. I stood in the hall momentarily with my eyes closed as I imagined the scene in the room. My heart pounded so forcefully that I could see little pulsations of light reflected off the insides of my eyelids. I tried to breathe deeply, but my chest was tight as if bound by a straitjacket.

Euphemisms Confuse Rather Than Comfort

I stepped in the room to see the little girl lying next to her mother in the hospital bed, crying and gently hugging and lovingly stroking her mother's body, which was pale and dusky and had already begun to stiffen. The family friends, who remained in the corner crying, spoke primarily Spanish but could speak enough English to let me know that they were close friends of the patient and were taking care of the little girl while her mother was in the hospital. I spoke to them first, but the little girl was in the room, so she could hear the conversation. I learned that she was in kindergarten, was very smart, and was bilingual. We weren't trying to hide anything, but I was trying to find out more about what others had told her. They explained that the nurse and doctor told them that the mom died and that the little girl was aware that her mom had cancer. They weren't sure if she really understood what cancer or death meant but shared that she was smart, outgoing, friendly, and very nurturing of her mother.

The clinical nurse leader offered to introduce me to the girl because she had already built a relationship with her. She said, "I want to introduce you to a friend of mine. Sujin works at the hospital too, and she wants to help you understand what happened to your mom. Would it be okay if she talks to you?" I asked the little girl if I could sit next to her while she continued to hug her mom, and she agreed. I knelt next to her at the side of the bed and said, "I'm so sorry that your mom died." I used the word *died* intentionally because in these situations, I find that adults have a hard time saying *death* or *die*, words that they think sound harsh and perhaps cruel. Many adults will instead use euphemisms like "Your mom went to be with God," "Your mom is now an angel," or "Mom is in Heaven now." I can appreciate that impulse because I was also tempted to use softer language to lessen the blow as I witnessed this child's obvious pain, confusion, and fear. However, euphemisms often confuse children, so I purposely used concrete language. My first priority was to educate the girl about death and the physical and biological changes that happen after death. This process can be very difficult, especially if others have confused the child.

Sometimes they cannot understand why mommy left them, or why God chose to take mommy away, or when mommy is coming back from heaven. They wonder, "When can I visit Mommy in Heaven?" We try to educate parents before death about how important it is to say *dying* and *death* to minimize misunderstanding, even though these words seem harsh and, for many adults, are difficult to say aloud.

After I said, "I'm so sorry your mommy died," she replied, "I know she died," while still crying. I then sat by her side in silence for a few minutes and said, "I know you're really sad. I know it really hurts. It's okay to cry." After a while, her crying eased and the room was quiet. I thought her crying may have been more a reaction to everyone else in the room than it was a genuine expression of grief because children at that age don't fully grasp the finality and permanence of death and therefore do not always demonstrate grief or sadness immediately. All the adults around her were very upset and continued to mourn quietly, and I think, at some level, she understood that something big had just happened. I started to explore her level of understanding by asking, "Do you know what happens to a body when somebody dies?" I think she responded that the body was sleeping, which is a very typical answer for kids her age. Then I said, "Yes, I know it looks like she's sleeping. But this is different from sleeping," and then I started my typical spiel: "You know when a body dies, it stops working. When our bodies are alive, we need to breathe, drink water, and eat food. We can move, and we sleep, and we talk." I listed the many things that living bodies do and continued, saying, "When a body dies, it does not need any of those things anymore because it doesn't work anymore." She thought about my words for a moment and said, "So my mom's body is broken."

I was surprised by her words because she seemed to be processing the information more than I expected for someone her age. I asked her, "Do you know what made her body stop working?"

"She was sick. She had cancer."

"Do you know what cancer is?"

"No."

"Cancer is the name of the sickness that your mommy had, and she was getting medicines to try to make the cancer go away. But the medicine wasn't working, so the cancer in her body got bigger and got into all different parts of her body. That is how the cancer broke your mom's body, made it stop working, and caused her body to die." She considered my words again for a moment and repeated, "So my mommy died." I just kept repeating, "Yes. Your mommy died. It was the cancer that made your mommy's body stop working and die. There was nothing that you did that made this happen." In addition to the goal of initiating understanding of death for this little girl, I also wanted to emphasize that she did not cause her mother to die as young children often have the misperception that they made things happen due to developmentally appropriate egocentric and associative logic.

Despite my efforts to help her grasp the situation, she reverted to covering her mother's body with the blanket and saying she thought her mommy was cold. Then I repeatedly validated her nurturing by saying things like "You took such good care of your mommy, but I want you to know that because her body has died, she doesn't feel cold anymore so you don't have to worry about covering her with a blanket, but you can if you would like to." Then at one point, she said, "I think my mommy is hungry," and proceeded to put crackers in her mom's mouth. As the little girl strained to reach up from the side of her mother's bed, someone else entered the room to see if we needed anything. I think it was a nurse assistant. When she saw what was happening with the crackers, she became overwhelmed with emotion and walked back out of the room with the patient's friends. Every few minutes, someone from the unit—a nurse, chaplain, unit clerk, or social worker—entered the room to offer help. Each one surveyed the scene silently from the foot of the bed for a few moments and became so overwhelmed by the sight of the little girl trying to tend to her mother that they left the room. I fought back the intense urge to cry as I envisioned my daughter trying to feed me crackers while I lay cold and still on my deathbed. I quickly reigned in my emotions because I knew I needed to fish the crackers out of the dead woman's mouth with my fingers before continuing to educate the little girl: "You know when a body dies, it does not feel hungry or need food anymore. You are so sweet and so loving to worry about your mom being hungry, but I want you to know that she doesn't feel hungry anymore, so you don't have to worry about feeding her." We continued to cycle through this process of education about the concrete meaning of death. She was holding her mom's hand and noticed that they were cold, so I again explained that when the body dies it stops working and turns cold but that she need not worry because her mommy did not feel cold. Then I said, "If it makes you feel better, we can put a blanket on her," because I felt that it was still important to her to comfort her mom.

The most challenging aspect of meeting this little girl was feeling very emotional myself. I found it incredibly difficult to be real and human and allow tears to roll down my face while still doing my job. I ultimately found it impossible to block out my emotions, so I forged on through tears. Just when I started to feel somewhat relieved that the little girl was beginning to understand what death meant, she would do something like try to open her mom's eyes and say, "Mommy, open your eyes. I need you to see me again." I had to keep reminding myself that kids usually need a while to truly grasp death while repeatedly reinforcing the message that "when a body dies, it cannot smell, or see, or hear." Despite my inner voice of reason and my determination to do my job, I could not control my emotions, and I eventually surrendered and grieved along with this child.

I was in the room with her for over an hour during which I followed her cues. At one point, she said, "I want to go for a walk." I thought that was a good idea, but I paused because during the pandemic, we were discouraging family members from walking around the hospital. I wasn't sure if walking around would be okay, but I felt as though she could use a break from the room. When we left the room, she said, "I need you to carry me," which was not surprising. Many young children demonstrate regressive behaviors when they become overwhelmed or stressed. I said, "I can't carry you because we are supposed to wear masks to stay safe from the germs in the air, but I can hold your hand." As she and I walked hand in hand down the hallway, we soon encountered a patient escort who was rolling a patient down the hall as she slept on the gurney. When the little girl saw them approach, she yelled, "Oh, that patient is dead too," which visibly alarmed the escort as well as other staff members who happened to be within earshot. Then I reiterated my earlier message by saying, "I know it looks the same, but that patient is actually sleeping," and we walked on. That brief scene confirmed for me that she was still appropriate for her developmental stage and that she was still trying to make sense of her mother's death.

A short time later, a man who was unrelated to the patient but who served as medical power of attorney arrived on the scene, at which point the little girl enthusiastically hugged him. She seemed okay, which was another sign that she was coping in a healthy and developmentally appropriate way because kids her age will cycle in and out of grief. Children process and cope through play, so I encouraged her to spend time with the many staff members who wanted to help her by entertaining her and playing with her. I then waited for her next cue. Someone found some children's books, so I sat down in a family room and read a little bit of a story that had nothing to do with medicine or her mother's death. Then she asked to see her mom again, so we returned to the room. She wanted to hug her mom and fix her hair, so I encouraged her to do so. After I had spent about two hours with the little girl, she said she wanted to return to the family room, so her mother's friends accompanied her there. Before she left, I repeated how sorry I was that her mother died and normalized her experience, saying, "I know you are going to feel sad. I know you are going to be scared, and that's okay. Your aunt will be here soon. I want you to know that you can share with your mommy's friends and your aunt and talk to them when you're feeling sad because I don't want you to feel sad by yourself." She was very bright and said that she understood. Then she asked, "Can I talk to you again today if I need to?" I told her, "Of course. Just let any of the nurses know you want to talk to me, and I will come back." She seemed happy and excited to go play in the family waiting room. I gave the patient's friends my contact information and asked them to share it with the patient's sister when she arrived. I also reviewed the signs of complicated grief in children so they could share this information with family and friends. They were wonderful and very supportive and loving of this child. They even took notes, wrote down my name and number, and promised that they would share this information and keep in touch with the little girl after they went back home. They wanted to honor their friend by helping support her daughter. Finally, I educated the two friends about how to use unambiguous language when speaking to the girl about death and shared that she will most likely continue to go back and forth between seeming to understand that her mother died to needing to be reminded again. Then the friends took her to the family room to hang out for a while. I think the friends started to feel better after they saw the child behaving like her outgoing, happy self again and grateful to be able to assume a role in her healing process.

Tending to the Healthcare Team

After the little girl left, I found the nurse who cared for the patient that day, a nurse's aide who cared for her the day before, and the clinical nurse leader to check in with them because I got the sense that several people were traumatized by this event. Of course, anyone who works in a cancer center knows that patients sometimes die in the hospital, but no one had witnessed a death with a young child present. I wanted to make sure that they understood that it is normal from the developmental standpoint for a four-year-old child to repeatedly vacillate between seemingly understanding that her mother was dead and then displaying a lack of understanding by trying to open her eyes, talk to her, feed her, and tend to her.

One of the nurses said that she had never been in a situation where a patient's child had come to the hospital. She said, "I didn't sign up for this, I am here to work with adults." She was not trying to be harsh; she just meant that she was not prepared for what had just happened. She described how terrible and helpless she felt, not knowing what to do for the child. The other nurse also said she felt helpless and added, "I have a little girl about the same age as the patient's daughter and I could not stop thinking about my daughter when I saw the little girl." They asked me what I told the girl so they would know how to respond if they ever found themselves in this situation again, so I summarized my meeting and emphasized the importance of using clear, unambiguous language when explaining death and allowing children time to process and grieve. The three nurses were young, so this may have been their first exposure to death. I think what motivated me the most that day was my hope that the little girl had a good head start understanding what happened to her mom so that by the time she reached the appropriate developmental age, about age 5 to 7, she would better understand the irreversibility of death, especially if the adults around her reinforce the message and nurture her emotionally. My hope in working with children who have the unfortunate experience of a parental death is that they will remember our interaction as empathic and nurturing. I want to minimize the trauma of such a significant loss at such a young age. My second priority is supporting the clinical team.

Closure

Just after the woman died, the nurse leader took a picture of the little girl holding her mother's hand, which she framed and mailed to the patient's sister after they returned home. A few months later, the family photographed the little girl holding that picture and sent it back to the team, who immediately displayed it prominently in their break room. Now, whenever the nurses feel sad at the memory of that day, they can look at the picture of the little girl wearing a bright yellow dress with her dark wavy hair pulled back into a ponytail, squinting into the afternoon sun with a big smile on her face.

PRACTICE POINTS

Key Reflections

- Hospital deaths are often extraordinarily stressful for patients, families, and members of the healthcare team. When a young child is involved as patient or survivor, stress levels rise exponentially.

- Adults who witness death, grief, or other intense suffering often do not know how to respond and therefore can feel utterly helpless. Those feelings of helplessness are heightened when a child is involved.

- Young children do not fully grasp the permanence of death until about age 5 to 7, so younger children often vacillate between expressing grief following the death of a loved one and displaying behaviors that would otherwise be considered normal.

- Feelings of grief and sadness are normal for clinicians whose jobs regularly expose them to death and other human suffering.

- One of the great challenges for clinicians who regularly witness suffering is performing their jobs skillfully and professionally while maintaining humanity and authenticity. Crying on the job is normal sometimes.

Empathic Actions

- Sometimes simply being present by sitting silently at a grieving person's side is the most powerful expression of empathy.

- When speaking to young children about sensitive topics, clinicians should use unambiguous language, such as *death*, *dead*, and *die*, rather than euphemisms, such as "Your mommy went to Heaven." Euphemisms confuse young children and can lead to feelings of rejection if they believe parents chose to leave them to go to heaven.

- One of the highest priorities for clinicians who speak to young children about death is to educate them about the physical and biological changes that death entails.

- Simple acts like holding a child's hand while taking a walk or reading a children's book for a few minutes can offer great comfort to a grieving child by providing an emotional break and an opportunity for developmentally appropriate play.

Empathic Expression

- "I'm so sorry that your mom died."
- "I know you're really sad."
- "I know it really hurts."
- "It's okay to cry."

- (Exploration) "Do you know what happens to a body when somebody dies?"

- "Yes, I know it looks like she's sleeping. But this is different from sleeping. When a body dies it stops working. When our bodies are alive, we need to breathe, drink water, and eat food. We can move, and we sleep, and we talk. When a body dies, it does not need any of those things anymore because it doesn't work anymore."

- (Exploration) "Do you know why she was sick?"

- "Cancer is a sickness that your mommy had, and she was getting medicines to try to make the cancer go away. But the medicine did not work, so the cancer in her body got bigger and got into all different parts of her body. That is how the cancer broke your mom's body, made it stop working, and caused her body to die. You did not do anything to make her sick or make her body stop working."

- "You took such good care of your mommy."

- "I want you to know that because her body died, she doesn't feel cold anymore, so you don't have to worry about covering her with a blanket."

- "If it makes you feel better, we can put a blanket on her."

- "You know when a body dies, it does not feel hungry or need food anymore. You are so sweet and so loving to worry about your mom being hungry, but I want you to know that she doesn't feel hungry anymore, so you don't have to worry about feeding her."

3 Safe and Empathic

 Approach to Opioid Use through the Lens of a Palliative Care Physician

Joseph Arthur and Daniel E. Epner

I THINK MUCH of my empathic ability is rooted in my upbringing in Ghana, a country in West Africa where I was born and lived until I moved to Pennsylvania for my internal medicine residency. My mother was an elementary school teacher, and my father worked as the manager of a shipping company, so I grew up in a stable middle-class home. My dad was a good provider, but he traveled extensively for work, so my mom was the glue that held our family together. Being a teacher, she emphasized education above just about everything else and assigned me additional schoolwork at home. As a result, my siblings and I all pursued higher education and professional careers in Ghana, the United Kingdom, or the United States. I was steered toward medicine from an early age, as many of the best students in Ghana are. My parents knew I had the potential to succeed as a doctor. In addition to being steered toward a medical career, I also naturally developed a great interest in medicine that intensified as I witnessed the difficulties that many Ghanaians experienced in seeking health care.

Life in Ghana and the political system there are relatively stable, unlike some other African nations, where ethnic and religious tensions breed violence and fear. Most Ghanaians have reliable access to food, shelter, and public education. However, life there is not nearly as affluent as the average US life, particularly concerning health care. Ghana has a universal health care system that has evolved extensively over the past several decades. In the 1980s, the government began the "cash and carry" system, which required Ghanaians to pay out-of-pocket fees at each point of service. This system excluded many people in the lower and middle classes who could not afford the fees. In the early 2000s, the ruling government launched the national Health Insurance Scheme, which provided universal health care to all Ghanaians for about 6% of the gross domestic product. Nonetheless, health care remains variable throughout the country, with urban areas having greatest access to hospitals, clinics, and pharmacies and rural areas having little or no modern care. Patients in rural areas still either rely on traditional African medicine or travel great distances for care. As I grew up and attended medical school in Ghana, I witnessed these inequities, which shaped my approach to medical practice.

First- and Third-World Problems

One of the things I remember most about medical school was caring for patients with sickle-cell disease, an affliction common to Africa that causes bone pain and pain in solid organs due to sticking of blood in small vessels. Sickle-cell patients in Ghana suffer tremendously because they do not have access to good pain medication. In fact, opioids are almost nonexistent in

Ghana and in most other developing nations for cultural, social, and political reasons. When I was in medical school, the strongest analgesic I could prescribe was pethidine (Demerol), which is not a particularly good opioid and one that we rarely use now. We managed our sickle-cell patients primarily with acetaminophen and nonsteroidal anti-inflammatory drugs. Having essentially no access to morphine or opioids during medical school, I naturally had little practical knowledge of pain management when I started residency in the United States.

I soon realized that this knowledge gap put me at a tremendous disadvantage at my large residency program, where many patients sought care primarily to address uncontrolled pain. Those patients had pain for myriad reasons, but a sizable proportion had sickle-cell disease. I was amazed by the contrast between management of pain from sickle-cell disease in Ghana as compared to the United States. In the United States, patients with pain had access to a variety of opioids in seemingly unlimited supply, and during my residency, many of my sickle-cell patients took multiple types of opioids in high doses. Nonetheless, many of them still experienced poor pain control, and they often visited the hospital repeatedly to access intravenous opioids. This paradox confused me: How can US sickle-cell patients experience such poor pain control despite ready access to opioids? I began to realize that pain perception is highly subjective and heavily influenced by many factors other than tissue injury. Pain is a complex construct accentuated by negative emotions, such as fear and anxiety. In addition, a significant proportion of patients with ready access to opioids, particularly in the intravenous form, take them for reasons other than pain, such as to experience euphoria. Many pain management experts refer to this phenomenon as "chemical coping" or high pain expression. Given the complexity of pain management, I had considerable practice prescribing opioids during my residency and therefore became relatively comfortable with the basic pharmacology.

The Complexities of Pain Perception

I later moved to MD Anderson Cancer Center in Houston for my hospice and palliative care fellowship. During my training, I quickly learned that opioids were the mainstay of cancer pain management, so I would have to become even more facile at prescribing them safely and effectively in all their different forms and doses than I was during my residency. Coincidentally, I read a lot about the opioid crisis in the United States and the increasing number of deaths related to it. Most of our cancer patients were legitimately taking escalating amounts of opioids for intractable pain. However, a sizable minority were taking excessive amounts of opioids out of proportion to their pain syndromes, physical findings, and imaging. This became evident to the whole team, including doctors, advanced practice providers, nurses, and the psychosocial team. While I was in fellowship at MD Anderson, a few of the faculty members in my department took a special interest in many aspects of pain management and started to develop research and clinical programs that focused on safety, effectiveness, and pharmacology. They found that we could identify patients as having high risk of aberrant opioid use by using validated screening instruments, including CAGE-AID (Cut down, Annoyed, Guilty, Eye opener—Adapted to Include Drug Use), SOAPP (Screener and Opioid Assessment for Patients with Pain), and the Edmonton Symptom Assessment Scale (ESAS).

A Wake-up Call

Shortly after joining the faculty in palliative medicine at MD Anderson, I cared for a 36-year-old woman with breast cancer who made an indelible impression on me and confirmed my commitment to developing safer and more effective treatments for pain. Her life was difficult even before she developed cancer, since she was the single mother of a 16-year-old daughter, her only child, and was therefore practically a child herself when she gave birth. She was somehow able to extricate herself from an abusive relationship with her daughter's father, and she lost contact with other family members. She was essentially isolated, barely scraping by financially, had little support from her community, and did not belong to a church. Fortunately, her widely metastatic cancer was responding very well to chemotherapy. From our standpoint, she was doing well with good pain control on a stable dose of short-acting opioid, which she took only a few times per day as needed for bone pain.

Then one day when she presented to our clinic for a routine visit, she was despondent, crying inconsolably from the moment she arrived. She explained that her daughter had recently overdosed on her pain medicine despite the fact that the child was seemingly healthy with no known history of anxiety, depression, or mental illness. Listening to her describe her profound guilt, grief, and sadness was heart-wrenching for everyone. She felt guilty for spending so much time away from home for treatments, never present to guide or encourage her daughter. She also felt guilty for having left her medications out in the open rather than securing them in a safe. She never dreamed her daughter would get access to them. Now she faced the reality that she would never share in the joy of important life events, like her daughter's high school graduation or marriage, and she would never hold a newborn grandchild in her arms. She also grieved the loss of everyday simple pleasures, like eating dinner with her beloved child or hearing her gossip about boyfriends or school cliques. She longingly remembered the many times when she would brush her daughter's hair as they sat on the couch watching a silly television program before bedtime. She never fully appreciated how precious those moments were until they were gone. The woman's life appeared black: meaningless and hopeless.

The Power of Presence and Support

When I saw her in the examining room, I was at a complete loss for words. I knew I should say something empathic, like "I am so sorry for your loss," but I found myself just sitting by her side in silence for several minutes as she continued to sob. I handed her a box of facial tissues and continued to sit there. She eventually regained her composure, at which point I quietly said, "I can see how much you loved her." I told her about options where she can get help in the community to guide her through her grief and made sure she had our contact information. We also explained methods for securing her opioids under lock and key. I then asked her to stay in the room to meet with our counselor, and I quietly left. After I did, our counselor returned and spent over an hour with her. Throughout the conversations with our nurse, our counselor, and myself, she assured us that she did not intend to harm herself. Through our intensive work during that visit and many subsequent phone calls and clinic visits, she gradually began to adapt to life without her daughter. We made it clear that we would stay by her side as she dealt with her grief and would consistently be a source of support for her. She was doing much better when we saw her later.

My experiences with this young woman imbued me with a deep sadness. Coming from a relatively poor country in West Africa, I was saddened to see people die unnecessarily in such a rich country as the United States, the great land of opportunity. Deaths during the opioid crisis are such a waste of human potential. As I thought more about her, my sadness turned to anger, which became determination to develop better and safer ways of caring for patients in pain.

I know I was not to blame for the death of my patient's daughter, which was instead the result of a perfect storm of psychosocial hardships that were set in motion long before I met her. Thankfully, my colleagues and I have made great efforts to create detailed patient education materials for safe opioid use, storage, and disposal and to establish safe practice standards for our clinic. We now advise all patients to keep their pain medications under lock and key, and we monitor them closely by phone and in person if we sense increased risk of aberrant opioid use or unsafe practice. I may not be able to prevent all future opioid-related injuries and deaths, but at least I can sleep at night knowing I am doing everything in my power to minimize them.

High Pain Expression

Another patient who made an indelible impression on me and who heavily influenced my approach to opioid management was a 65-year-old man who had developed severe pain due to side effects of radiation and chemotherapy for head and neck cancer. We appropriately prescribed escalating doses of pain medicine for the few months of treatment and for several weeks after he went into remission. However, we became concerned when his opioid requirements remained high, and he continued to express high levels of pain even after his skin and oropharynx had healed completely months later. In our clinical judgment, he should not have required opioids so long after recovery. Yet he remained on a 75-microgram fentanyl patch and took hydrocodone/acetaminophen 10/325 mg tablets six times per day for breakthrough pain, and he often presented to clinic claiming to have taken even more than six breakthrough doses on many days. As a result, he often ran out of hydrocodone tablets earlier than he should have and requested early refills. His opioid regimen corresponded to more than 200 mg of oral morphine per day even though he appeared completely healed from the side effects of treatment. Of course, we could not know how he felt, but we ultimately concluded he was using pain medicines for reasons other than to treat pain.

This situation and others like it create great discomfort for our palliative care team, as they undoubtedly do for many others, because we pride ourselves in practicing compassionately and always giving patients the benefit of the doubt. We practice what Carl Rogers termed unconditional positive regard, which is the basic acceptance and support of a person regardless of what the person says or does. Our success depends on our ability to forge healing relationships with our patients and their families. Nonetheless, we knew we would have to confront this man in a compassionate way if we were ever going to taper his opioids.

Setting Limits Is Necessary Sometimes

After delving a bit deeper into his medical history, we learned that he had an underlying substance use disorder that had existed long before his cancer diagnosis and that he had been in a rehabilitation program multiple times for alcohol and recreational drugs. I reviewed the Texas Prescription Monitoring Database and noticed that he received a prescription for 80 hydrocodone tablets from a provider in his community a few days before his most recent clinic visit, even though we told him repeatedly that only one team should prescribe his pain medicines and that we were that team. His random urine drug screen collected a few weeks ago also showed the presence of marijuana and oxycodone in addition to the fentanyl and hydrocodone we prescribed. The database did not show a prescription for oxycodone within the past two years, suggesting that he had obtained the oxycodone from someone other than a healthcare provider. In addition, there were no telephone notes or messages in his electronic record documenting that he had tried to reach our clinic team with questions or concerns. He was often manipulative or antagonistic during previous visits with only a doctor present in the exam room, so I anticipated tremendous resistance when I attempted tapering his opioids.

Stay Calm and Carry On

I took a deep breath and closed my eyes for a few seconds as I disinfected my hands in the hallway outside his room. I thought our conversation would be tense at best and hostile at worst. I reminded myself not to take negative language personally or let Mr. S. throw me off my game, which is always to put the patient's interest first.

After the usual pleasantries, I asked Mr. S. if I could review the prescription-monitoring database and recent urine drug screen results with him, and he replied, "Sure, knock yourself out, Doc."

I pulled my chair around beside him so we could review the report together and said, "I am concerned by some of the things I see on your prescription record." I then pointed at the most recent entry on the report. "I noticed you got a prescription for hydrocodone a few days ago from Dr. X on the north side of town."

"Doc, I was hurting, so he gave me a prescription, but I never picked it up."

"Perhaps someone picked it up for you, because the record shows it was filled."

"I don't think so. I don't know who would have picked it up, but I don't have it. Do you want me to call my wife to see if she picked it up?"

I considered letting him call his wife, but I sensed he was creating a smokescreen that would send us on a long tangent. I knew I would need to stay on task to avoid letting him wear me down. I decided to ignore the question and move on. He had succeeded in diverting me from asking more about the inappropriate hydrocodone prescription. I continued:

"You said you went to Dr. X. because you were hurting, but I don't see any telephone encounters or messages in your medical record that showed you tried to contact us."

"All I know is that I tried to call this clinic a bunch of times, but no one ever picked up the phone or called me back."

I decided to confront him as gently as possible: "I am surprised to hear that, since our nurses are very reliable about answering the phone or at least returning messages within a few hours."

Our conversation then took on a more threatening tone:

"Doc, are you calling me a liar?"

I quickly ran through various responses in my head. I thought he was lying, but I did not want to antagonize him by saying so. I decided to return to first principles, which is to always make the patient's needs our top priority: "All I know is that we want to take care of you the best we can. These medications can be harmful, so we want to make sure you are taking them safely and that no one else in your household is at risk."

He then turned up the heat: "Doc, I know where you're going with this. I hate all these questions. You are the only doctor in this clinic who speaks to me like this. You're talking to me as if I'm a criminal and you think I'm getting high with these meds and selling them. I want a different doctor."

I would normally feel a sense of failure if a patient threatened to fire me, but in this case, I was hopeful that he would actually do so. Nonetheless, I knew I could not get off the hook that easily by passing this challenge on to one of my colleagues. I was determined to stick with him and make some real progress before he left. I tried some education and empathy: "I hear you're frustrated. I know it must be hard to hear these questions repeatedly, but we want to make sure you are using your pain medications safely and getting the most benefit from them. I get worried when you take more pain medication than we prescribe for you or run out of your medications early. We are having this conversation because we care about your safety and the safety of those around you."

My honesty seemed to disarm Mr. S briefly, perhaps because he had difficulty remaining angry with someone who truly cared about him. Nonetheless, he was determined to get what he came for. He paused for a moment and then said, "You don't know how I feel. I may not look like I'm hurting, but I have a high pain tolerance. I need meds."

I next replied with four empathic phrases followed by a dose of reality: "I can't possibly know how you feel. I realize you are suffering. Your situation now is different than it was before. I know it seems like I'm being punitive, but I really just want to take good care of you and make sure we use these medications safely. Our job is to relieve as much of your suffering as possible to help you live as well as possible." I tried to demonstrate through my actions that sometimes doing the right thing is unpopular and more difficult than acquiescing.

At that point, he went on an intricate and lengthy tangent: "Doc, the pain I am feeling now reminds me of the time I got into a motorcycle accident 30 years ago. No, maybe on second thought it was 34 years ago. Yes, I had just come out of the service and returned stateside and was traveling back to Nebraska when my bike slipped on the ice. Then an eighteen-wheeler came along. ... I fractured several vertebral bodies and ribs. ... Was hospitalized in the ICU for several weeks...I have very high pain tolerance, did not even need opioids then, but this pain I am experiencing now, this pain is ten times worse!" As he droned on and on, I felt as though he was trying to manipulate me, wear me down, and distract me. I listened politely as long as I could tolerate it and then stood up and said, "Please excuse me. I will return in a few minutes with some other members of the team to develop the best plan for you."

Sometimes a Team Approach Is Necessary

I have to admit it: I felt frustrated by what I perceived as Mr. S's attempts to manipulate me into renewing his opioids prescriptions at their current levels. Doing so would have been the path of least resistance, would have allowed me to see other patients more quickly, and would have gotten me home earlier. I knew my wife would be upset if I showed up late for dinner again. We have an 11-month-old daughter, our first child, and we want to be present for her. Nonetheless, I realized I had a job to do, and deferring that job to the next visit would only embolden Mr. S and place him and those around him at increased risk. I composed myself for a moment outside his exam room, walked to the workroom where other doctors, nurses, and counselors were typing and talking, and assembled other team members who could help me formulate a plan.

Over the past few years, colleagues in my department and I have developed an interdisciplinary team-based approach to compassionately care for patients like Mr. S who demonstrate aberrant behaviors related to opioids. These behaviors include using more pain medicine than prescribed without consulting us, not using prescribed pain medications (as evidenced by urine drug screens) but asking for refills anyway, repeatedly running out of pain medicine early, obtaining opioids from multiple prescribers, using recreational drugs, verbally abusing nurses and other members of the team, missing scheduled appointments repeatedly without rescheduling, and dropping into clinic unannounced to demand refills, often moments before the clinic closes. We call our approach Compassionate High Alert Team (CHAT), which includes the doctor, the nurse, the pharmacist to offer patient education, a patient advocate, a counselor to provide psychosocial support, and an armed police officer on the very rare occasions when we feel physically threatened.

This interdisciplinary team approach allows us to establish ground rules for safe opioid use, builds trust in patients, and helps them feel supported and cared for. In addition, when multiple team members are in the room together, patients are not able to pit one member of the team against the others or manipulate the doctor by changing the medical history on a whim. The doctor usually leads the conversation, but other team members are available to contribute when necessary. This coordinated approach projects a sense of confidence and cohesion. The presence of three or four members of the clinical team creates a power imbalance and therefore can make the patient feel intimidated. However, such a power imbalance helps the team set healthy boundaries and limits, which protect the safety of patients who thrive on structure, something they may not have experienced before.

My approach to the conversation depends on the situation. I usually ask the nurse to notify the patient before the whole team enters to normalize the situation. During the visit, we acknowledge the fact that opioid use disorder is a condition that can be managed just like any other disease and validate the patient by saying that we know the pain is real, if I truly believe it is. We also try to be as transparent as possible and avoid beating around the bush. However, on the rare occasions when I strongly suspect but do not have proof that the patient is using pain medicine solely to create euphoria or to divert to other people, I do not usually say so explicitly. I always stress that safety is our first priority.

Prebrief

The CHAT team convened and debriefed with everyone in the workroom before going back to see Mr. S. I summarized the medical history briefly in plain language for the patient advocate, who is not a clinician, and then explained my rationale for calling everyone together for the meeting:

> Thank you for being here to help develop the best plan for Mr. S, who was treated with radiation and chemotherapy for head and neck cancer but who is now fully healed. We are concerned by what we perceive as excessive use of opioids so long after recovering from therapy with no evidence of recurrent cancer. He has a history of substance use disorder, so he is at high risk of aberrant behaviors and has displayed several such behaviors in recent weeks. Our entire team, including nurses, pharmacist, and I, all think we should taper his opioid regimen, but he is resistant.

I next explained the strategies I planned to use for the conversation:

> I want to warn everyone that this conversation at times may feel uncomfortable and may even become

confrontational. Please remember we are having this conversation with Mr. S's best interests in mind. Of course, I will follow the same exploratory and empathic paradigm we all use every day, by asking the patient for his perspective and responding empathically when emotional moments arise in the conversation. I will try to let him speak as much as possible. However, I may have to redirect the conversation if he goes off on tangents or appears to be manipulating us. Is everyone comfortable with this strategy?

At that point, everyone, including the patient advocate, nodded yes and expressed no concerns. The nurses were relieved that our team was finally having a frank conversation with Mr. S, because they were frustrated by their interactions with him in recent weeks. The patient advocate was also comfortable with the approach because she had seen so many similar encounters that she was confident in our skills, judgment, and knowledge.

Compassionately Setting Limits

The three of us entered the room to meet Mr. S. Of course, we intended to be supportive, but we realized that he may have perceived the meeting as intimidating or confrontational. I therefore began by addressing this issue: "Mr. S, I brought other members of the team to help us develop the best plan for your pain management. I know it may feel intimidating to have all of us here at one time, but Ms. C is here to advocate for you, and the pharmacist is here to help with medication related questions you or I may have."

The advocate and pharmacist then introduced themselves, after which Mr. S smiled amicably. I became optimistic, because I thought he would be on his best behavior in front of multiple witnesses. I continued: "Now that your mouth and throat sores have healed, I feel strongly that we should reduce the size of your fentanyl patch with the intention of tapering off all opioids within a few months." My optimism was apparently premature because after he contemplated my suggestion briefly, he said, "I can't believe you are pulling the rug out from under me! It's always the same with you people! You are treating me like some kind of junkie. I'm no drug addict! I really hurt!" He then resumed his lengthy tangent about the events around his motorcycle accident many years before, his high pain tolerance, the withdrawal symptoms he developed when they stopped the pain medicines suddenly last time, and many other peripherally related issues, all in dramatic fashion.

I again listened silently for as long as I could, just as I had during our original conversation, and then intentionally interrupted him. I formed the letter T with my hands like football referees do when they signal "time out" and said, "I want to take a time out for a moment to refocus this conversation." He kept talking over me, at which point I said, "I really need to reenter this conversation because we have listened carefully to your concerns and now I need a chance to address them." He continued to speak, at which point I had to be more assertive and firmly repeated, "No, now it's my turn." He finally stopped talking, so I continued: "I can tell you have many valid concerns, so I want to address each of them one by one." I felt as though we were finally getting somewhere because Mr. S had shared his fear of withdrawal and uncontrolled pain, even though he had done so in an exasperating fashion. In addition, he was listening to me at least momentarily and, by sharing his concerns, had opened a door for empathy.

I continued: "It sounds like stopping pain medicines last time was very difficult for you. The whole ordeal must have been miserable. I promise we will help you through this process and be available to you. We are on your side. We will taper gradually and steadily. However, for us to succeed, you have to do your part. If at any point we think you need to see an addiction specialist, we will do our best to help you identify one."

His face and body relaxed a little, but he nonetheless offered another show of resistance: "I still don't think I'm ready to go down on the fentanyl."

I remained steadfast: "Yes, I am confident you are. This is a very good medical plan, so let's stick with it." He seemed resigned to the fact that we were not going to back down, and he may have finally realized that we were on his side, so he lowered his head silently in tacit agreement. We reduced the 75-microgram fentanyl patch to 50 micrograms and instructed him to continue hydrocodone for breakthrough pain no more than four doses per day. We then suggested he return one week later, at which point he said, "Oh, Doc. I can't come back up here every week! The drive here takes an hour each way, and I spend $15 just to park each time. I can't afford the gas, let alone the parking." I was never under the illusion that this conversation would be easy. I knew tapering off opioids would be an incremental and emotionally draining process, so I suggested a two-week follow-up instead. He replied, "Doc, can't we just make my appointment in a month?" I again felt compelled to seize control of the conversation and avoid being manipulated because I worried about him going home with a full month's supply of pain medicine. He finally agreed to return in two weeks, and over the ensuing few months, our team was able to taper his opioids. The process was stressful at times, because Mr. S occasionally tested us by reverting to aberrant behaviors, but he generally stuck with the program.

My Golden Rule of Patient Care

My daughter is learning to walk, mostly cruising around the house leaning on tables, chairs, and walls but sometimes taking a few awkward steps on her own. Yesterday was a beautiful spring day, unseasonably cool for Houston, so my wife and I took our daughter to the park in her stroller. She usually loves to play on the slide and swing, but city workers had cordoned them off with yellow tape due to the coronavirus pandemic.

I entertained her the best I could by holding her in my arms as we chased ducks and jogging around with her on my shoulders. Yesterday was not her birthday or some other momentous occasion. It was just an ordinary day in the park, much like countless days I hope to enjoy with her as she grows up. Nonetheless, my experiences yesterday with my family were profoundly important and precious to me. On days like yesterday, I mourn the loss of my patient's daughter who died of an overdose, and I say a silent prayer: "God, please protect my baby from harm, keep her safe, healthy, strong and resilient as she grows to be a woman. Guide her to make good choices." Days like yesterday provide perspective to help me see clearly that my job as a physician is to protect my patients from harm as I protect my family.

I know that my relationship with my daughter will have its difficulties as she grows up. She will undoubtedly pout when we forbid her from driving around town with friends in the wee hours of the morning or if she does not work hard in school. My wife and I will be upset if she ever behaves disrespectfully or takes her comfort and privilege for granted. We know we will have to set limits at times because young people need limits and guidance to flourish and grow, even as they gradually gain their independence. Patients also sometimes need guidance and limits. I will always respect my patients' autonomy, but I will be there to guide them compassionately with my knowledge, skill, and experience. My golden rule is to treat my patients as I would a beloved member of my own family.

PRACTICE POINTS

Key Reflections

- Pain perception is highly subjective and heavily influenced by many factors other than tissue injury.

- Pain is a complex construct accentuated by negative emotions, such as fear and anxiety.

- A significant proportion of patients with ready access to opioids, particularly in the intravenous form, take them for reasons other than pain, such as to experience euphoria. Many pain management experts refer to this phenomenon as "chemical coping" or high pain expression.

- Aberrant behaviors related to opioids include

  - using more pain medicine than prescribed without consulting the healthcare team;

  - not using prescribed pain medications (as evidenced by urine drug screens) but asking for refills anyway;

  - repeatedly running out of pain medicine early;

  - obtaining opioids from multiple prescribers;

  - using recreational drugs;

  - verbally abusing nurses and other members of the team;

  - missing scheduled appointments repeatedly without rescheduling; and

  - dropping into clinic unannounced to demand refills, often moments before the clinic closes.

- Sometimes setting limits with patients and establishing healthy boundaries is the most empathic and safe strategy.

Empathic Actions

- When someone is grieving, sometimes the most empathic thing to do is to simply be present and say little or nothing.

- Clinicians who prescribe opioids should give patients detailed education materials that describe safe opioid use, storage, and disposal and establish safe practice standards for their clinics. For instance, they should advise all patients to keep their pain medications under lock and key.

- Clinicians also need to monitor closely patients who take opioids, especially if they sense increased risk of aberrant opioid use or unsafe practice.

- Clinicians can identify patients as having high risk of aberrant opioid use by using validated screening instruments, including CAGE-AID, SOAPP, and the ESAS.

- An interdisciplinary team–based approach to compassionately caring for patients who demonstrate aberrant behaviors related to opioids allows the healthcare team to establish ground rules for safe opioid use. Such an approach builds trust and helps patients feel supported.

Empathic Expression

- Patient says, "Doc, I know where you're going with this. I hate when you people ask all these questions. You're talking to me like I'm a criminal and you think I'm selling my meds."

  - Traditional response:

    - "No one ever called you a criminal."

  - **Recommended empathic response:**

    - "I know it is hard to hear these questions repeatedly, but we want to make sure you are using your pain medications safely and getting the most benefit from them. I worry when you cannot accurately describe how you use your meds and you sometimes take them in ways that are different from how we pre-scribe them. We are having this conversation because we care about your safety and the safety of those around you."

- Patient says, "You don't know how I feel. I may not look like I'm hurting, but I have a high pain tolerance. I need these medications."

  o Traditional response:

    ▪ "I am just trying to do what is best for you now."

  o **Recommended empathic response:**

    ▪ "I cannot possibly know how you feel. I realize you are suffering. Your situation now is different than it was before. I know it seems like I am being punitive, but I really just want to take good care of you and make sure we use these medications safely. Our job is to relieve as much of your suffering as possible to help you live as well as possible."

- Patient says: "I can't believe you are pulling the rug out from under me! It's always the same with you people! You are treating me like some kind of junkie. I'm no drug addict! I really hurt!"

  o Traditional response:

    ▪ "No one called you a drug addict. However, I think it is time to stop these pain medicines. You do not need them anymore."

  o **Recommended empathic response:**

    ▪ "It sounds like stopping pain medicines last time was very difficult for you. The whole ordeal must have been miserable. I promise we will help you through this process and be available to you. We are on your side. We will taper gradually and steadily. However, for us to succeed, you have to do your part. If at any point we think you need to see an addiction specialist, we will do our best to help you identify one."

- Patient says, "I still don't think I'm ready to reduce the fentanyl."

  ○ Traditional response:

    ▪ "Yes you are. I know you can do it."

  ○ **Recommended empathic response:**

    ▪ "I know you are worried about reducing the dose, but I am confident you are up for the challenge. We made a good plan together and our team will be here to support you throughout this process."

- Patient says, "I've been giving my son some of my pain medication."

  ○ Traditional response:

    ▪ "You should never share your medications, and your son should take only what we prescribe for him in the way we prescribe it."

  ○ **Recommended empathic response:**

    ▪ "You are sharing your medications because you cannot stand to see him suffering like this. If he were my kid, I might do the same thing. I can tell you really love him and will do anything for him. Having said that, I think we can do an even better job taking care of his symptoms, and we think it is important for you not to share medications with him."

- Patient says, "I've been coming to this clinic for two years, and every doctor has given me the meds I need. You are the first doctor who has denied me."

- **Key Concept: Oftentimes, empathy should be tempered with a dose of reality:**
  - "Your situation now is different than it was before. I know it seems like I am being punitive, but I really just want to take good care of you and make sure we use these medications safely."
- Patient says, "I am afraid I will become addicted."
  - Traditional response:
    - "Many people worry about that, but I doubt you will become addicted. Let me explain the difference between addiction and tolerance."
  - **Recommended empathic responses:**
    - Provider: "I can see why you are nervous about that. Tell me more about what worries you."
    - Patient: "My daughter is addicted to dope and has been in jail a few times. I finally had to break off ties with her. I am raising her 2-year-old daughter."
    - Provider: "It sounds like you are going through a real rough patch. It must be hard to see your daughter suffer like that, and I am sure you are suffering too. Have you ever used recreational drugs?"
    - Patient: "No, I have always been a teetotaler. I rarely even drink alcohol."
    - Provider: "Great, then your risk of addiction is very low. Let me explain the difference between addiction and tolerance, which is a normal response to pain medication."
- Patient says: "Weed is the only thing that helps. I smoke five times a day."

- Traditional response:

  - "Marijuana is illegal and unregulated. We do not want you to mix marijuana with pain medications. In fact, we cannot prescribe pain medications if you continue to smoke marijuana."

- **Recommended empathic response:**

  - "I do not blame you for doing everything you can to get by. Cancer is not easy. Having said that, I think we can do a better job of controlling your symptoms than you can with marijuana. In addition, I am concerned marijuana will not mix well with your other medications, like pain medication."

- Patient says: "I got this weed from a state where it's legal, so it is regulated."

  - Traditional response:

    - "Marijuana is illegal in Texas, so I cannot recommend using it. I could lose my license if I prescribe opioids for you."

  - **Recommended empathic response:**

    - "I do not have a moral stance on using marijuana, and I realize it is legal in many states. However, I am concerned about potential side effects between marijuana and your other medicines like your pain medicines. We want to work with you to taper off marijuana to the extent possible."

4 | A Son's Duty

Ahsan Azhar and Daniel E. Epner

THE MANY TIMES I practiced chest compressions and mouth-to-mouth resuscitation on CPR mannequins for basic life support (BLS) recertification, I never imagined the surreal experience of performing CPR on my own mother, in her bedroom, in front of other close family members. I have never served in combat, but I can now imagine the flashbacks experienced by those who have witnessed the horrors of war. Memories of that day in my parent's home sometimes jolt me like an electric shock during conversations about goals of care with my patients and their families on the palliative consult service. One such conversation remains fresh in my mind from just a few weeks ago.

Uncomfortable Silence and Vexing Questions

The patient was a man in his 50s with relapsed, refractory leukemia whom the oncologists were trying to guide toward a comfort care route since he had exhausted all treatment options for his leukemia. The treating team asked us to assist with this transition and to manage symptoms. The patient and his family were all from the Indian state Punjab, which borders Pakistan, my parent's home country, so I am fluent in their native language, Punjabi. The patient was delirious and therefore unable to communicate more than very rudimentary information, and his wife spoke only Punjabi. As a result, the patient's wife deferred all substantive communication to their young adult son, who was fluent in Punjabi and English, having studied and worked in the United States for several years. They had a daughter as well but she lives in India with other family members. The situation placed a tremendous burden on their son, who was to participate in all communication with the healthcare team and make many important decisions on behalf of his father.

Before I entered the room for the first time, I debriefed with the bedside nurses, who explained that the family was very emotional and overwhelmed. The son was seemingly upset with the quality of his father's care, but he was in fact grieving his father's impending death and was having difficulty expressing his grief. As a result, he often came off as passive and was sometimes even a bit surly. I thought this young man might be having difficulty communicating with female staff, so I hoped to be able to connect with him better. After introducing myself in Punjabi and explaining my role, I asked how we could help the patient feel better, looking back and forth between the patient, his wife, and their son. The patient was deeply delirious and minimally responsive, and his wife was silent despite the fact that I addressed her in her native tongue, so I turned my gaze to his son. He was silent for several seconds and then responded in English "Why is my dad not eating? What can you do about it?" I replied, "I know how badly you want to nourish your father so he can regain strength. I can only imagine how difficult it is for you to see him in this weakened state." I then paused, at which point, the son said, "But we need to feed him or he will die! How can he recover without food?" I then tried a slightly different strategy, mixing empathy with a clear medical explanation in an attempt to help the son understand. "I wish we had better options for him, but his body is so ill now that it is no longer able to use nutrients even if he were to ingest them. His lack of appetite is due to his body shutting down. This is part of the dying process." I then waited for a while to see what would emerge, yet the son remained withdrawn and silent, so I asked, "What are you thinking about? Would you mind sharing your thoughts?" He sat in silence for several seconds, at which point I offered more empathy by saying, "I respect how strongly you are advocating for your father. You carry a huge load on your shoulders. I know your mother is counting on you to make all major medical decisions for your father, and I can imagine that must be overwhelming for you, especially at such a young age." I thought this barrage of empathic expression would draw him out of his shell and encourage a much-needed and cathartic crying spell, but he remained dispassionate. I had made every effort to connect for over 30 minutes by giving him room to express himself and by expressing empathy, yet he still refused to open up.

When India and Pakistan were partitioned several decades ago, the province of Punjab split down the middle, with predominantly Muslim citizens settling in Pakistan and people of other religions settling in India. Although tensions between the two countries remain to this day, I was confident that my background had nothing to do with my inability to connect with the patient's son. For one, I introduced myself and started speaking Punjabi without telling them that I was from Pakistan. In addition, the patient and his family were Sikh, and I have never felt any religious or cultural tension between Sikhs and Muslims during my interactions. As a result, my Muslim background, even if they had been aware of it, would almost certainly not have been a source of tension or awkwardness. Furthermore, my perception is that Sikhs are generally very peaceful, loving people. This is a generalization, of course, but I understand that the Sikh ritual leaders often speak about peace, harmony, and kindness. Therefore, cultural issues did not explain the distance between us. I could see that I was not making much ground there and when I asked if there was something we could offer, he declined and politely asked me to leave.

"Doctor, What Would You Do If He Were Your Father?"

When I returned the next day, I met the son in a separate room. I again tried to connect with him by asking a few open-ended questions in an attempt to get him to express himself, yet he continued to rebuff me, responding with at most single-syllable words. I felt that I might have been able to connect better if he were older, since nearly all of my patients are older. I am not sure whether my feelings of discomfort around teenagers and young adults result from my own insecurities or whether they reflect a true lack of connection, but young adult family members often seem to have little to say to me during my visits. After a few more minutes of silence, he finally asked, "Can you help us get the new treatment for his leukemia from India? We have been waiting for weeks for it to arrive, but it is held up by travel restrictions related to the Coronavirus pandemic." He was referring to an Ayurveda herbal remedy that a family friend from home recommended to treat leukemia. I thought the chance that an herbal remedy would appreciably inhibit leukemia growth was essentially zero, but I did not say so; instead I said, "I respect how hard you are fighting for your dad. I also respect how hard he has fought his illness over the past several months. I know this entire ordeal must be incredibly stressful for you and your family." He again brooded in silence for a few minutes and then asked, "Doctor, what would you do if he were your father?"

Career Evolution

As the young man posed this question, I flashed back to the image of my mother lying in bed as I tried to resuscitate her.

After a few seconds, my thoughts turned to memories of my father and mother who came to the United States in their youth so that my father could develop his career as a pharmacist after he completed his pharmacy degree in Pakistan. Being an only child, my mother was the true picture of a sandwich generation, caring for both her parents and her own family. I was born in the US but moved to Pakistan when I was very young. Fortunately, my dad made every effort to visit us once or twice a year. I tell myself now that I did not feel much of a void not having my father around during those early years in Pakistan, but I am probably kidding myself. I am sure I longed for his presence, but my memories of that time are hazy. I do remember writing letters and sending them by postal mail, since there was no email at that time. Our family also often traveled back and forth between the US and Pakistan, especially during summer vacation. I even have fond memories of our grandmother accompanying us to the US on one of those visits. However, when it came time for college and career development, I returned to Pakistan. We had family support there, and school was much less expensive. That is how I became an international medical graduate, even though I spent a good part of my childhood in America. Hence, throughout my life, I have had the opportunity to view both cultures extensively.

As soon as I completed my medical degree, I immediately returned to the USA for residency, since all the best programs were here. When I went through residency, the closest thing to palliative medicine I saw on the inpatient wards was geriatrics, since geriatricians sometimes came to our noon conferences to join the conversation. During residency, I worked on a research project that focused on the palliative needs of patients with advanced gallbladder cancer. This was in 2001 in the immediate post-9/11 period. I interviewed many cancer patients during the few months that I worked on that research protocol and got to know a lot about their symptoms and the difficulties they experienced. I am not sure why I decided to help with that particular research project, but the limited exposure I got from it was my first real taste of palliative medicine, although I had not yet heard the word "palliative" at that time.

After completing residency and my initial board certification in internal medicine in the US, I decided to return to Pakistan for my first job, responding to an advertisement for an internist to work in a cancer hospital there. However, the job required knowledge of palliative care. At first, I figured that I did not have the necessary experience, because at that time I lacked formal palliative medicine training. However, after thinking a little more, I concluded that I can meet the requirements because of my participation in the palliative/oncology research project during residency. The people who interviewed me must have agreed because they offered me the position without hesitation. My job involved working beside many subspecialists, such as gastroenterologists, oncologists, and pulmonologists, who started to send me all the patients who they thought were no longer candidates for aggressive, disease-directed therapy, such as cancer patients who could no longer tolerate chemotherapy. There were many such patients, and the subspecialists had neither the time nor the expertise to manage their symptoms or engage in conversations about goals of care and transitioning to a comfort strategy, since they carried such heavy clinical loads. I had no formal communication or palliative training at that time, but I learned on the job through trial and error. That is how I started developing more interest and skills in palliative medicine, even before my palliative fellowship. My journey to a career in palliative medicine followed a winding path rather than a paved highway.

When the Boundary Between Doctor and Son Blur

While I was working in Pakistan in that first post-residency job, the boundaries between my work and my family lives were blurred when my mother became severely ill back in the US. She suffered from complications of heart disease, diabetes, and a chronic lung ailment; she developed pneumonia and spent weeks in the hospital and several days on a ventilator in a US hospital. I was able to get coverage for my clinical duties in Pakistan, so I left my family for several weeks to be at her bedside. Her doctors told us she was not going to make it, so my dad called my brother and me from the US to ask whether he should start thinking about a scenario under which the doctors would ask us to take her off the ventilator. My father's question got me thinking about many related conversations I had with my mother when I was a young adult. My mother in some respects made conversations about her goals and priorities easy because she would not address questions head-on in any detail. She would say, "When the time comes, we will deal with it." On the other hand, I remember her giving me hints about how she may have wanted to approach the end of her life, casually during regular conversations, almost in passing. For instance, she told me, "I hope to die peacefully in my own bed. I hope and pray that I do not linger at the end." I also gained additional insight from opportunities to accompany her to visits paying her respects to friends and relatives over the years when someone got sick or died or to celebrate significant life events. I was essentially her chauffeur for many such excursions and was able to eavesdrop on her conversations. After some of these condolence calls, while she and I drove back home, she would say that the decedent had "died so miserably" and "that experience must have been so distressing for the family. I hope our family does not have to go through such an experience." Listening to her as we drove around town gave me tremendous insight regarding her philosophy of life and priorities, even though she did not complete an advanced directive. Despite my mother's desire to die in her own bed, when she became acutely ill, she opted for aggressive care and ended up on the ventilator. Fortunately, she gradually improved and got off the ventilator, so we as the family did not have to decide whether to withdraw it. After this long ordeal, she recuperated for many weeks and made it back to her home in the US. At that time, my grandmother was living with me and my nuclear family in Pakistan. My mother always told us that she wanted to be at home with her mother and children at the time of her death, so she returned to Pakistan after several more months of rehabilitation and recuperated well over the next 2 years.

I was out of town attending a course when I received a call from home that my mother's condition had suddenly worsened due to an upper respiratory infection that progressed to pneumonia. Despite the gravity of her situation and underlying frailty, my mother refused admission for intravenous (IV) antibiotics. Instead, she wanted to return home to do the best she could with oral antibiotics. She never spoke about code status in the hospital or after returning home. She told me, "I'll be fine." Despite her reassurances, I hurried back home from the city where the course was held.

A Missed Opportunity for a Gentle Caress

My mother was still doing fine on the evening of my arrival, and we were able to have time together, but her condition deteriorated rapidly. Knowing how tenuous she was, my grandmother maintained a near-constant vigil at my mother's bedside so my wife and I could watch our young children. Late in the evening after my return, my grandmother summoned us anxiously from my mother's room. When I entered, I saw my mother lying still and silent, eyes partially open, pale, and breathless. In the few moments it took me to absorb the shocking scene, I became paralyzed with indecision, stuck in an awkward limbo between doctor and son. As a well-trained and skilled doctor, I was supposed to know how to save sick patients. Yet, this was no sick patient lying before me, but rather my beloved mother! My grandmother stood silently against the wall, as if she was trying to give me a wide berth to perform a miracle, yet I wondered what she actually expected of me: revive her daughter or respect her daughter's dignity? Which hat should I wear: doctor or son? Ultimately, my doctor instincts took over. As my grandmother looked on anxiously and my wife kneeled at my mother's side, I reflexively started CPR, rhythmically compressing the same chest from which I breastfed as a baby. Mercifully, my attempt at resuscitation lasted only a few minutes, because I soon accepted the fact that my mother was gone. Many months later, my wife told me, "You knew your mother was gone, but you still continued resuscitation for a while." I said, "You're right. I think I was just trying to help my grandmother by showing her that we at least tried something." When I recall that day, I often wish I had instead kneeled by my mother's side, caressed and kissed her forehead, and held her hand. I wish I had held my grandmother in a silent embrace to comfort her through her worst nightmare rather than performing CPR on her daughter.

What Do You Think He Would Want?

As I stood lost in my memories, my patient's son repeated his question: "What would you do if he were your father?" His question awakened me and returned me to the scene in his father's hospital room. I quickly reoriented and said, "Yes, a very difficult question: What would I do?" As I surveyed the scene, I again felt so sorry for the poor lad who carried the weight of his family's unrealistic expectations on his delicate shoulders. He was in his mid-20s, but he was still a child in many respects. He desperately needed someone to relieve his onerous burden. I considered recounting the story of my mother to help him reach a decision about his father, but I decided against it. Our circumstances were so different. I instead asked, "What do you think your father would want now if he could tell us? How would he want to live at this point?" He sat silently for several seconds and then said, "I do not know what he would want. I barely knew him." His voice wavered slightly as tears began to well in his eyes. I paused and said, "Tell me more about that." He explained that his father traveled most of the time for business when he was a child, so the two spent little time together. When his father returned from long trips, he often spent time alone in his study reading the paper or watching television. When he was midway through high school, his parents sent him off to an elite prep school in America to seek a better life. Before leaving for the US, the boy had not spent even a single night away from home. He loved nothing more than to hang out with his older sister and her friends, listen to pop music, gossip about schoolmates, and watch Bollywood movies. Then his parents suddenly sent him halfway around the world to live in a dormitory full of American boys who taunted and bullied him for his foreign-sounding name and lack of athletic prowess. As the young man spoke, I imagined the depths of his loneliness. He survived the indignities of high school by building a hard shell around his heart to wall off his feelings and ultimately gained admission to a selective American university as his parents demanded. The boy felt guilty for complaining about his circumstances because he knew his parents wanted the best for him, but he soon resented the responsibility of carrying his family's reputation on his shoulders.

I listened for several minutes and said, "It sounds like you never got the chance to know your father. You have fended for yourself from an early age." At that point, he described the one special occasion he shared with his father, on his 7th birthday, when just the two of them spent the entire day admiring exotic animals at the zoo, riding roller coasters at the amusement park, and eating special treats from street vendors. As he recalled that cherished memory, he turned away from me in an attempt to hide the tears streaming down his face. We stood in silence for a few minutes until he turned toward me again. I said, "None of this is your fault. You have displayed incredible courage through this horrible ordeal. No one should have to make such difficult decisions for a parent." I wanted desperately to tell him unambiguously to let his father live his final days in peace rather than focusing on medical issues. However, I instead expressed my recommendation in the form of a question: "Do you think your father would want to focus on his comfort and dignity at this point? He has fought so hard and suffered tremendously, but he still has his dignity." I think my question spoke volumes because, for the first time, the boy seemed decisive and confident. He replied in perfect Punjabi, so his mother could understand: "Yes, I think it best to focus on my father's comfort and dignity. He has fought bravely, but now is not the time to offer more chemotherapy. We need to respect his humanity."

As he spoke, my thoughts returned to my mother, but this time not on her deathbed as before. Instead, she sat beside me in the passenger seat of our car as we drove through the countryside en route to congratulate friends on the birth of their first grandchild. My mother wore a long flowing pashmina across her shoulders that fluttered in the fresh spring air. The shawl was deep green, like the verdant forest surrounding us, inlaid with delicate gold fibers that glistened in the sun as it fluttered in the breeze. My mother's face radiated health and beauty again as she smiled broadly and told me how happy she was to meet the newborn baby and welcome new life into this world.

PRACTICE POINTS

Key Reflections

- Trauma from our personal lives can influence our medical practice, just as trauma from our medical practice often informs our personal lives.

- Medical professionals often find themselves caught between the role of being a caring and supportive family member and the role of being a skilled and compassionate healthcare provider.

- Often when patients or family members are subdued or not communicative, their silence reflects strong negative emotions lurking beneath the surface, such as sadness, grief, fear, and frustration.

- Family members can feel overwhelmed when given the responsibility to make life-or-death decisions on behalf of a gravely ill patient, especially when linguistic barriers exist between the healthcare team and the patient.

- People from different cultures, geographic regions, and religions are more alike than they are different.

- When young physicians follow their interests and passions, they are very likely to develop career paths that best suit their aptitudes and skills.

Empathic Actions

- Debriefing with other members of the healthcare team and carefully reviewing the medical record before a challenging conversation helps one to get in the right frame of mind and to develop a strategy for the conversation.

- Sticking with patients and families even after they rebuff us by repeatedly making ourselves available is a powerful way of saying, "I care."

- One of the most important and difficult tasks of any compassionate physician is to have honest and sensitive conversations about prognosis and goals of care with their patients, especially those who face serious illness.

- As difficult as it is to discuss goals of care with patients, it is arguably even more difficult to do the same with members of one's own family.

- When a patient's family member asks "What would you want if he were your father/mother/child?" the best approach is an exploratory one:

  ○ "What do you think your father would want now if he could tell us?"

  ○ "How would he want to live at this point?"

Empathic Expression

- "I know how badly you want to nourish your father so he can regain strength. I can only imagine how difficult it is for you to see him in this weakened state."

- (Empathy followed by important biomedical information) "I wish we had better options for him, but his body is so ill now that it is no longer able to use nutrients even if he were to ingest them. His lack of appetite is due to his body shutting down. This is part of the dying process."

- "I respect how strongly you are advocating for your father. You carry a huge load on your shoulders. I know your mother is counting on you to make all major medical decisions for your father, and I can imagine that must be overwhelming for you, especially at such a young age."

- "I respect how hard your father has fought his illness over the past several months. I know this entire ordeal must be incredibly stressful for you and your family."

- "None of this is your fault. You have displayed incredible courage through this horrible ordeal. No one should have to make such difficult decisions for a parent."

5 | My Soul Is Bleeding

Marvin O. Delgado Guay and Daniel E. Epner

Dr. Delgado is a geriatrician and palliative care specialist whose scholarly focus is spirituality and religion in supportive and palliative care.

Know Your Own Soul

Growing up in a very observant Catholic household in Guatemala, I lived only a few blocks from the church, so I sang in the choir and my family attended mass every Sunday. We all knew the friars well. I became so involved in Catholicism that I felt a true calling from God to enter the seminary. However, I was torn because I knew from a young age that I also wanted to be a doctor. Regardless of whether I became a priest or a doctor, I knew my main calling was service to others. My family and I often visited patients in the hospital and taught others to read and write. I asked my priest, "Should I be a priest, or should I be a doctor?" He never pushed one way or the other, but he told me, "Whenever you awaken in the morning, ask God 'what do you want me to do with my life?'" I kept that phrase in my mind as I deliberated over time, after which I concluded that I could best serve others by becoming a doctor. At that time, I thought I could cure illness and still attend to patients' spiritual needs. However, I now know that illness is often incurable, and that spiritual distress can be as tenacious as a wine stain on white linen. Nonetheless, I am glad I chose medicine because it challenges me every day. I do not participate in religious rituals as much as I used to, but prayer remains an important part of my life and I still maintain a strong connection with God and my faith. Clinicians need to know themselves and be in touch with their own souls to be able to touch another person's soul, which is not easy. My response to losses and happiness in my life reflects who I am. I thank God for being alive every single moment. In my mind, it does not matter how bad things may be in my life because when I am with a patient, I need to do my best to help him.

Opening a Spiritual Door

I saw a patient in his mid-60s in the palliative care unit while on call one weekend who expressed pure existential and spiritual distress in the face of death and suffering. He had advanced cancer that was no longer treatable, and he was receiving high doses of painkillers and anxiolytics. He was a widower after his wife died two years before. In fact, he told me that she died in the very same room that he then occupied. He did not say so explicitly but dying in the same room where he tended to his wife in her final days must have added even more trauma to his life. He was treated with antidepressants and anxiolytics during the last five years, but he never had a history of suicidal ideation. Nothing in his electronic record documented any discussions of spirituality or spiritual distress.

Before the hospitalization, he was living with one of his two adult daughters who cared for him and devoted herself to him, although he was alone when we met. I sat in a chair next to him as he lay in bed. I said, "How are you doing, how was your night?" The first thing he said was, "This pain is horrible, and I cannot stand it anymore. My pain is unbearable." After he said that, I sat in silence for several seconds to see what he would say next. "I just cannot withstand this pain. It is horrible." I asked, "Is your pain physical or some other type of pain?" He looked at me for a while, started crying, and said, "I just don't know." I said, "I would like to know more about your pain. How is your spirit doing?" He considered my question in silence and then said, "I cannot withstand this pain. I feel as though my soul is bleeding. My soul is hurting." "Tell me a little bit more about the pain that you feel in your soul." He had rated spiritual pain as six on a scale of 10 on the symptom inventory, which is high, so I knew there was something else besides the physical pain. Then I asked him again to tell me more about the pain in his soul, and he repeated "I just feel like my soul is bleeding."

One of my passions outside of work is creating brightly colored art, so when he spoke of his soul bleeding, I imagined that everything around us was bleeding, like red rain running down the outside of the window during a rainstorm. At that moment I thought, "Oh my God, all the pain medicine and anxiolytics in the world will not relieve this man's suffering." So, I waited for him to say something else about the bleeding, and after a while he said, "I just can't stand it anymore." I asked, "Are you experiencing fear or worry that is making your soul bleed so hard?" He said, "I don't know what will happen to me after I die." I asked, "Is there anything you do that gives you strength or peace to work through all this?" He cried at times, which I took to be a healthy, cathartic process, and other times he was quiet. I just sat with him in silence, allowed him to regain his composure after he cried, and listened as he resumed talking. Later, he acknowledged that he was not able to achieve peace of mind about the future, and I assured him, "We will continue to help you any way possible to achieve peace in your soul."

I realized that my compassionate presence and silence were the most healing things I could offer him because at a sacred moment like that, he was allowing me to be present. It must have been very hard for him to open his heart in front of me, someone he had never met before. I believe I created a connection and established an environment where the patient felt safe to express himself fully.

Spiritual Teamwork

Then our conversation turned to religion. He said, "I don't know. I think I need to offer my confession." He then mentioned something about being baptized again, at which point I asked, "So how was your relationship with God before you got sick?" He told me that his connection with God has not always been great and God has not been present in his life recently. "I suffered a lot when my wife died and drifted even further from God." "Do you think that strengthening your connection to God will help you now?" "Yes, I think I may feel better than I do now if I reconnect with God." So, I asked, "Is there anything else that we can do to help you get more connected with God?" "I guess you can pray for me. Then perhaps I will confess my sins and get baptized."

I am a physician, not a spiritual adviser, so I do not have the training to know how to delve more deeply into someone's past traumas, guilt, and shame. I think involving the psychosocial and spiritual team in these circumstances is very important. I told him, "Okay, we work as a team. I have a chaplain on my team who I can ask to visit you, and I can also help you connect with your own pastor or spiritual leader if you want." "Yes, I have not been to church much lately since my wife died, so that would be helpful." I then explored a bit more about his relationship with his family and how his children interacted with him after his wife's death. There must have been something deeper about their relationship that was affecting him. He initially did not say anything when I asked about his family, but I did my best to do a life review, finding out what he enjoyed doing with his family and friends. After a while he appeared more peaceful and said, "Okay, let's just take one day at a time," and I assured him we would help with his physical symptoms, emotions, and connection with God to give him as much peace of mind as possible.

Later that day, I talked to our chaplain who was able to contact the patient's pastor, and both visited the next day. I never knew what the source of his distress was, but I think he needed to offer a secret confession about an event in his life many years before that did not involve his family but that profoundly worsened his existential distress. After attending to his spiritual needs, we were able to decrease his pain medications and anxiolytics substantially. After a few more days, he went home with one of his daughters to enter hospice. His daughters remained involved in his care until the end. They spoke with the chaplain and pastor frequently, because they needed the opportunity to tell the patient they loved him and were sorry, which helped him feel much calmer. After his death, his daughters called the unit a couple of weeks later to thank us for caring for him so well and for helping him achieve peace. He only lived a short time after I met him, but he was able to achieve at least some measure of peace in his soul by expressing his distress.

We clinicians sometimes feel as though we do not have control over anything when we cannot fix medical issues. Of course, dying is no picnic. Nonetheless, we can decrease suffering profoundly with our presence, even without medications and other medical interventions. In fact, our presence is most healing under circumstances when we have the least to offer medically. I sometimes wonder what I am supposed to do or say when speaking with patients in distress, but then I realize my power is in being present and encouraging them to express themselves. I think the other lesson for me is that we clinicians need to be alert and listen for expressions of extreme distress so we can focus on someone's humanity rather than reflexively increasing pain medicines or anxiolytics when someone cries out for help. Facilitating expression about existential, spiritual, and religious topics is not easy. The easy part is adjusting the medications. We need to make time to sit down and explore the suffering to promote deeper healing. One of the most gratifying aspects of caring for the man in the Palliative Care Unit was that his spiritual advisors and I were able to dramatically improve his life just by allowing him to express his existential concerns and confess his sins. I was not qualified to receive his confession, but I was able to open the door to his spiritual life and let experts delve more deeply into specific religious and spiritual issues. My main role was to open that channel of communication because if I had not touched the spiritual side, nobody would have. Cultivating and nurturing my connections with patients and acknowledging their emotions and spirituality also helps me grow in my life and become a better doctor.

Opening a Spiritual Window

For me, exploring a patient's humanity and spiritual life is not a "one and done" process. After the conversation gets going, I often ask, "How are you holding up with everything that is happening to you?" or "How are you dealing with everything?" Frequently, if not always, I ask, "How is your spirit doing?" or "Do you have any spiritual or religious beliefs that help you walk through this process?" These simple open-ended questions open all kinds of doors, not just about religion and spirituality. Even people who are not religious usually seize the opportunity to respond by discussing anything important in their lives. I then continue to explore in a free-flowing way, adapting to whatever the patient says. The other very important question is, "What do you feel helps give you meaning in life?" because even people who have no religious beliefs experience their own spirituality. Many people consider their purpose in life and the things that give their life meaning to be sacred. So, it is important to explore spirituality in a general sense. I also ask, "How important is God in your life?" Some people say, "I believe in God, but God is not that important to me." They may say that their family or their work is more important than God. Others say, "God is the single most important thing in my life. Without God, I would not be here." Some people who experience a crisis say, "I used to have strong faith, but not anymore. After I got this cancer, I asked myself, 'What kind of God would allow this to happen to me?'" Identifying these attitudes and beliefs is important because they can be signs of maladaptive religious coping that affect how we care for the patient. Another question that allows us to connect is, "Are you part of any religious or spiritual community that helps you work through all this?" I do not ask about any particular religious denomination. Then I can find out more about their specific rituals. Sometimes I say, "I am not familiar with your religion, so can you share with me a little bit more so I can learn?" The last question is, "How can we help support you in your spiritual life or any other way?" I always express my gratitude when people open up about sensitive issues, because those conversations are sacred moments. I feel a sense of peace, tranquility, and accomplishment when I connect with patients meaningfully to help them live better. Spiritual assessments should not be like scripts or kitchen recipes, but rather free-flowing conversations.

The Angel in All of Us

I was recently asked to speak about goals of care with a woman in her 60s whose condition was rapidly deteriorating due to COVID superimposed on advanced cancer that was no longer responding to treatment. Everyone involved in her care was distressed because she wanted to remain full code and be intubated and resuscitated even though her outlook was dismal. We talked about her illness and then I asked her about her relationship with God and how important God was for her. She started to cry as she shared with me her fear of death, and then, much to my relief, calmly said that she wanted to die naturally when her time comes rather than be resuscitated. As our conversation was ending, I asked whether she wanted to share anything else with me before I left. She thought for a moment and said, "I prayed to God to help me understand what was happening to my body and how I should live, and he sent an angel to talk to me to explain everything." At that moment I forgot how hard it is to witness gravely ill patients suffer every day. I shed the anxiety, fear, frustration, and fatigue that all clinicians experience. This woman's words supercharged my soul. Angels are spiritual beings believed to act as attendants, agents, or messengers of God who are conventionally represented in human form with wings and long robes. However, this woman told me that clinicians who listen generously, explore and respect their patients' spirituality, and support them during their darkest days can be real-life human angels.

PRACTICE POINTS

Key Reflections

- Empathic and compassionate clinicians and spiritual leaders have much in common since their work is built on a solid foundation of tireless service to others.

- Clinicians need to know themselves and be in touch with their own souls to be able to touch another person's soul.

- Being in touch with one's soul involves finding out who one really is beneath superficial appearances and defining the ideals one represents. Many people believe that the soul is nourished by meaningful relationships with other people, with the natural world, and with a higher power.

- Touching another person's soul involves respecting and supporting who they truly are and helping them cultivate meaningful relationships with others, with the natural world, and with their spirituality.

- Diagnosing illness and prescribing treatments is challenging but is nonetheless much easier than touching a patient's soul.

- Empathic practice is a team sport. When it comes to matters of spiritual and existential distress, clinicians serve their patients best when they facilitate collaboration with chaplains and other spiritual leaders.

- Clinicians need not be spiritual or religious themselves to explore and respect the spirituality and religious faith of their patients.

- Patients who experience existential or spiritual distress at the end of life often harbor deep-seated feelings of guilt or shame.

- Opening one's heart to another is an act of courage.

Empathic Actions

- Clinicians sometimes feel as though they have no control when they cannot fix medical issues. However, they can decrease suffering profoundly with their presence, even without medications and other medical interventions. In fact, their presence is most healing under circumstances when they have the least to offer medically.

- Compassionate presence and silence are often the most healing things a clinician can offer a patient who is experiencing existential suffering.

- Clinicians who establish an environment where patients feel safe to express themselves promote meaningful connection.

- Clinicians should be alert and listen for expressions of extreme distress so they can focus on a patient's humanity rather than reflexively increasing pain medicines or anxiolytics when someone cries out for help.

- Clinicians who cultivate and nurture their connections with patients by acknowledging their emotions and spirituality grow in their own lives and heal themselves.

Empathic Expression

- The following simple open-ended questions open all kinds of doors, not just about religion and spirituality. Even people who are not religious usually seize the opportunity to respond by discussing anything important in their lives. Spiritual assessments should not be like scripts or kitchen recipes, but rather free-flowing conversations.

  o "Tell me a little bit more about the pain that you feel in your soul."

  o "Is your pain physical or some other type of pain?"

  o "How is your spirit doing?"

  o "Is there anything you do that gives you strength or peace to work through all this?"

  o "How important is God in your life?"

  o "How was your relationship with God before you got sick?"

  o "Do you think that strengthening your connection to God will help you now?"

- ○ "Is there anything else that we can do to help you get more connected with God?"

- ○ "How are you holding up with everything that is happening to you?"

- ○ "Do you have any spiritual or religious beliefs that help you walk through this process?"

- ○ "What do you feel helps give you meaning in life?"

- ○ "Are you part of any religious or spiritual community that helps you work through all this?"

- ○ "I am not familiar with your religion, so can you share with me a little bit more so I can learn?"

- ○ "How we can help support you in your spiritual life or any other way?"

- Classically empathic phrases:

  - ○ "We will continue to help you any way possible to achieve peace in your soul."

  - ○ "I respect your strong faith. Faith is powerful medicine."

  - ○ "We work as a team. I have a chaplain on my team who I can ask to visit you, and I can also help you connect with your own pastor or spiritual leader if you want."

6 Sticking by My Patients, No Matter What

Isabella C. Glitza Oliva and Daniel E. Epner

I AM A medical oncologist who cares exclusively for patients with advanced melanoma, most of whom have brain metastases or leptomeningeal disease (LMD). I always start conversations with patients during our first meeting by asking them what they understand about their illness. By doing so, I get a sense of what they know, and where I have to spend more time explaining. I have found that one of the best things about Internet search engines is that they empower my patients to learn about their cancer, but at the same time, these same Internet search engines can offer a lot of misinformation and false hopes. For example, one of my patients recently replied, "Oh my god, I searched LMD on Google, and it was so bad, I turned the computer off immediately without reading further." However, this allowed me to pick up where the patient stopped reading, and to provide more understanding of their disease. Treatment for patients with metastatic melanoma and other malignancies has changed dramatically over the last decade, as we now have effective options, including targeted therapies and immunotherapy. These new agents yield responses that we could only dream of a few years ago while being fairly well tolerated. Now, many patients with metastatic melanoma live many months or even years, and we oncologists have all seen patients who were incredibly sick but rose like a phoenix when treated with these new agents. However, I work in a large referral center, so most of my patients come to see me for a second opinion after having already received all those novel therapies. These patients are definitely more challenging since I often cannot offer further treatment, which can be heartbreaking. For my patients with LMD, life expectancy is typically weeks to months, and one of my jobs is to develop novel treatments for patients with this cancer complication. As a result, I constantly face heart-wrenching conversations with my patients about whether to offer treatment for LMD or whether to forego treatment and pursue a purely palliative approach.

The Importance of Great Mentors in My Life

When I finished my internal medicine residency and started my medical oncology fellowship a few years ago, I had not yet charted a specific academic focus within oncology, and I certainly had not thought much about melanoma. I was unlike many of my colleagues who knew before starting oncology training that they wanted to focus on a particular highly specialized academic area, such as molecular biology research, gastrointestinal cancers, or experimental therapeutics. However, when I was on the one-month melanoma rotation, I worked with Dr. Nicholas Papadopoulos, who we affectionately called "Dr. Papa" or simply "Papa." Dr. Papa was a melanoma medical oncologist who practiced medicine before the discovery of effective therapeutics, when stage IV melanoma was essentially a death sentence for all patients, not just those with LMD. He offered chemotherapy to many patients nonetheless, like his colleagues who treated melanoma did, but this practice was in many respects palliative medicine masquerading as medical oncology.

When I worked with Papa as a fellow, we had just started to use ipilimumab, one of the new 21st-century immunotherapies that lead to durable responses in a small subset of patients. For our LMD patients though, we used interleukin-2, an old-fashioned immunotherapy, which Dr. Papa injected straight into an Ommaya reservoir leading to the spinal fluid. He had done this approach for decades, and while it had significant side effects, it actually led to "cure" in some patients. I remember thinking that this was the "coolest things ever," primarily because somebody actually took on the challenge of trying and had the passion to do something for these patients. Working with him made me realize that I wanted to subspecialize in the treatment of melanoma patients, with an emphasis on patients with LMD, as I realized that nobody would take over their care once Dr. Papa retired. Therefore, when I finished fellowship, Papa retired the same day and handed his LMD patients over to me.

I must admit, caring for patients with LMD is very challenging. Many LMD patients die very rapidly, despite my best efforts. Dr. Papa was one of the most compassionate and empathetic physicians I have ever met who was humble and took care of his patients with unparalleled passion and determination, and I wanted my work to carry on Dr. Papa's legacy and offer hope to patients who suffer from LMD. Dr. Papa was old school. He would burst into the patient's room, larger than life, and would announce enthusiastically, "You are my hero! Congratulations. Your scans look great!" He rarely offered significant details and spoke in a heavy Greek accent. When I was still a fellow working with him, sometimes patients would hold me back after he left the room and ask, "What did he say exactly?" This would always worry me, as I wondered how they would agree to a certain treatment without understanding their prognosis or the implications of receiving treatment. However, I also learned that while a good number of his patients did not understand all that he said, they seemed satisfied with the good news and usually asked few if any questions. In addition, it seemed as though his patients relaxed after seeing him, no matter how anxious they were before. Dr. Papa would not initiate a long conversation about prognosis, and strangely, his patients rarely asked. He would just say, "Let's try this next!" That was the end of the conversation most of the time. It made me realize that Papa's overwhelming positive aura comforted his patients more than any words could have. His patients simply trusted him to be there for them, regardless of what happened. His body language, facial expression, and aura were Dr. Papa's way of saying, "We are not going anywhere. We will stick with you no matter what." Dr. Papa did not have the same access to the great treatments that I have today, but he had a big heart and willingness to stick by his patients during their darkest hour. His particular communication style never backfired on him, but it sometimes backfired on me when I took over his practice after he retired. Most of his patients' cancers would progress, and I had the task of sitting with them to say that cure or even meaningful life prolongation was no longer realistic. I would qualify the lack of meaningful treatment options by saying that palliative support does not mean that we are giving up on them. However, I wonder how comforted those patients were by my reassurance. Most patients were not shocked to hear the news, but a few said they had never imagined their melanoma was incurable. I wonder whether those patients actually knew their melanoma was incurable but did not want to say it aloud. I learned a lot from watching Dr. Papa, and hope that I have been able to incorporate the best aspects of his communication style into my own, even if we have very different styles.

Dr. Suresh Reddy is another wonderful physician from whom I learned a lot about communication and end-of-life conversations. I spent six months paired with him in the supportive care clinic as my weekly continuity clinic just when

I started working with Dr. Papa. Dr. Reddy started his career as an anesthesiologist but transitioned to palliative medicine several years ago. I learned a great deal by watching Dr. Reddy and his colleagues in palliative medicine discuss goals of care and end-of-life issues with patients and their families. One of the things that impressed me most about Dr. Reddy was how he was able to direct his undivided attention to patients through verbal and nonverbal means that communicated, "You are all that matters to me at this moment." This seemingly simple skill helped him form strong bonds with his patients. After these 6 months with him, I advocated that all hematology and oncology fellows should spend more time working in the palliative care department, since helping patients navigate important decisions about their care, especially as their treatment options become more limited, is arguably the most important task of a good medical oncologist. I even considered seeking board certification in palliative medicine but ultimately decided against it due to time constraints, but I am always grateful for the care that colleagues in palliative medicine provide for my patients.

Honesty and Authenticity

I follow a few key communication principles. First, people need to feel that we are 100% present when we speak with them, which is the principle Dr. Reddy and Dr. Papa instilled in me. People also need to hear the truth delivered in a way that adapts to their needs. For instance, when patients seem overwhelmed, I usually navigate the conversation gently by posing a series of open-ended questions, including: "What do you know about your condition and where you stand now? Is there someone in your family who you want to receive sensitive information for you? Have you ever discussed what would be important to you and how you would want to live if treatments do not turn out as well as we hope they will?" In contrast, I am more direct with patients who seek specific biomedical information. I also have to be honest when patients run out of treatment options for their cancer. I acknowledge and validate their fear. I think that my patients rarely if ever hold the truth against me. I think this stems from the fact that they get to know me, and that they know I will never "abandon" them, even if I might have to say that we need to switch to supportive care or hospice. I often acknowledge from the beginning when presenting the initial game plan with all the different options that I do not have a crystal ball that will tell me how each of the potential plans will work out, but that I will be honest when the time comes to stop cancer treatment. So far, all of my patients have appreciated my honesty, even though the truth is often very painful. I struggle as much as my patients do to accept the fact that we have exhausted all treatment options.

Besides honesty, another quality that I think patients appreciate the most from their clinicians is authenticity. I try to be enthusiastic, like a cheerleader, for as long as doing so is honest. However, I also do not try to hide my worries and distress if I am uncertain about what the future might hold or if I can no longer offer disease-directed therapy. I never look forward to having such serious conversations, even though I have had them countless times. I even cry with my patients on occasion and sometimes offer a hug to those to whom I am closest. I think there is something therapeutic about displaying authentic emotion. Patients do not expect us to be robots. Revealing our humanity rather than always pretending everything is perfect is another way of showing that we care.

To Treat or Not to Treat?

For the majority of patients, my colleagues and I would easily agree on whether or not to offer treatment. However, we all meet the occasional patient for whom our emotions and our objective medical judgment collide. One such patient for whom I cared recently was a man in his late 30s from Europe who presented to MD Anderson for the first time in very frail condition, wanting to know if there was "anything left for him to try." His melanoma had progressed despite several lines of targeted therapy and immunotherapy, and the bottom line was that he was near death by the time he was admitted to our hospital to address several acute issues. When I met him and his wife for the first time as his new oncologist on the inpatient service, I wondered before entering the room how our conversation would go. The advanced practice provider who saw him earlier that morning briefed me that he was very sick, which confirmed my impression from reviewing his medical records. I decided to see him at the end of rounds when I could devote my full attention to him and not have to worry about all the other patients. I dreaded my first meeting with him during the minutes before I entered his room, since I was not sure if he and his wife had unrealistic expectations based on their exposure to marketing campaigns that touted miraculous cancer cures. I feared he and his wife had traveled here from abroad expecting a miracle even though he was too sick to receive treatment.

After much deliberation, I finally entered his hospital room. He was as debilitated as I envisioned, appearing almost skeletal, pale, and slightly somnolent. He wore a nasal cannula for supplemental oxygen and worked so hard to breathe that he was mildly sweaty, entirely naked except for the sheet covering his groin. I sat down next to him, and after the usual introductions and pleasantries, I asked him and his wife who sat at his other side what they understood about his condition: "Where do you think you are in your illness now?" He paused for a few seconds, perhaps disarmed by the abundant space I afforded him and his wife to express themselves. They seemed to expect me to get down to business immediately and offer a treatment plan. He then said, "I know I am very sick, but I came here to find out what other treatment options may be available."

As he spoke, I resumed an internal debate that has raged within me numerous times. According to evidence-based practice guidelines, his extreme frailty clearly precluded disease-directed therapy. I am well aware of the metrics that show how often patients receive chemotherapy inappropriately during their final 30 days of life. Then again, what is "inappropriate," and who decides? His melanoma had ravaged his liver, lungs, and other vital organs. Objectively speaking, he was simply too sick to tolerate cancer therapy. On the other hand, while his cancer had progressed despite many different targeted therapies and immunotherapies prescribed elsewhere, he had never tried traditional cytotoxic chemotherapy. I bounced back and forth between opposing positions like two lawyers arguing a case: Yes, he had never received chemotherapy, which rarely yields long-lasting benefits for patients with melanoma, but sometimes it can "buy time." Did he travel here determined to receive treatment for his cancer, or would he instead be satisfied not receiving treatment, knowing that he had turned over every stone? What should I recommend to this poor man and his wife who had traveled so far to see me? The most difficult part of my internal deliberations was the prospect of having to tell him and his wife that he is very likely to die here in the United States without making it back to see his family and friends in Europe, regardless of whether he received more treatment or not. In addition to being too frail to travel, he also faced travel restrictions imposed by the global coronavirus pandemic.

While I deliberated internally and tried to imagine what he really wanted from me, his wife spoke up: "What about trying chemotherapy?" I answered, "I am willing to try traditional chemotherapy, even though it is unlikely to help, or we can instead focus on your comfort. I will support you either way." After sitting silently to let this information sink in, I felt compelled to add, "Regardless of our treatment approach, I am very concerned that you will die far from home in the hospital." I felt as though I had crushed his hope with a sledgehammer. Explaining that he would almost certainly die in the United States far from home was all the more difficult because he was originally planning to see me in my clinic in a few weeks under stable circumstances. Beginning our relationship by saying, in essence, "You will die here soon and never return home" without having the chance to form a relationship with him felt cruel and abrupt. I felt like I had to adapt to this messiness in order to help guide his decision-making. This scenario felt like the relational equivalent of working in the shock trauma room in the emergency center, when someone needs to crack a patient's chest and clamp the bleeder.

After I told the man and his wife I would support him whether or not he decided to take chemotherapy, I hoped they would give me clear guidance regarding which direction they favored. I find that patients who have suffered tremendously are often receptive to the idea of stopping disease-directed therapy and are at peace with their impending death. They seem to realize that the only thing that they can still control is their ability to make decisions about how they want to live. They get to the point where they say, "I will just move forward and take it as it comes, one day at a time." In contrast, their family members may still be in the fix-it mode and push for more treatment, since cancer has taken away their sense of control. However, in this case, neither the patient nor his wife offered direction. They were leaving the decision to me.

I realized that they needed more time to weigh their options, so I recommended a brain MRI to evaluate for brain metastases. As I left his room after staying a bit longer to discuss the side effects of chemotherapy, I felt sad thinking how unfair his situation was. I also looked at the man and his loving, strong but desperate wife and wondered what I would want if he were my husband. I quickly decided that I would want to be as aggressive as possible, but also reminded myself that they are not me. After his brain MRI later that day revealed a four-centimeter metastasis that caused mass effect and pressed on his midline, I returned to share the news. I explained that chemotherapy was even less likely to work and could actually make him worse even more rapidly by reducing his platelet count and causing a massive bleed in his brain, even if it shrunk the cancer in his liver. I spoke to them about code status, and he signed the do not resuscitate (DNR) order at the same time he signed the consent for chemotherapy. As he handed back the chemotherapy consent form, he looked me in the eyes and said, "Dr. Glitza, I just need to know that I tried everything." I walked away from that conversation with goosebumps as I wondered how anyone could demonstrate such strength, composure, and dignity in the face of such profound sadness and impending death. He and his wife never screamed, cried, or yelled. They just said, "We understand." He ultimately received one cycle of chemotherapy and died a short time later from liver failure.

Deliberations for the Future

In retrospect, my interactions with this patient provide an example of how my colleagues and I sometimes struggle with offering additional treatments rather than gently switching the focus to comfort with a natural and dignified death. Interactions like these sometimes leave me shaken, because I have a close bond with a patient, or I want to honor a patient and family's wishes to receive more treatment, or because I see one of my family members in them. I believe that there is no "right" or "wrong" and that these decisions are complex. The decisions I face with my patients with LMD are particularly complex, since they present to me seeking additional treatment despite the fact that they were told, "you have a few weeks to live." LMD has such a dismal prognosis that hospice and experimental therapy are literally the only evidence-based approaches with the current state of the art. In addition, clinical trials often do not benefit individual patients as much as they advance the state of our knowledge for future patients. I realize that we sometimes find it difficult to stop cancer treatment even though in reality doing so is actually the farthest thing from "giving up."

How I Will Handle Similar Conversations in the Future

As difficult as it is to treat patients with advanced melanoma and LMD, I am beginning to realize that treating the cancer is ironically the easy part. Many clinicians can learn to prescribe chemotherapy, targeted therapy, and immunotherapy. The hard part is offering something truly therapeutic to those patients who cannot safely receive more cancer treatment. The key to doing so is empathy.

What would my conversation with the young European man and his wife sound like if I could do it over again? It would sound a lot like many of the thoughts I had but did not share with them. Upon seeing him lying in bed near death, I would have immediately told him, "I admire your fighting spirit. You have traveled a long way to seek better treatments after having already fought so hard at home." I would have then immediately turned to his wife, who miraculously transported him to our hospital under the dir-est circumstances, and told her, "I respect how much you love your husband. I would like to think I would do the same for my husband if he were sick." I can imagine how healing those words would feel to the man and his wife, even before any talk of che-motherapy. I would have asked the man and his wife what was most important to them. Perhaps he would have replied, "I came here to seek more treatment for my cancer, but more than any-thing else, I need to feel that I have done everything in my power to fight this disease, even if I eventually succumb to it." I may have then acknowledged that he needed to turn over every stone and then said, "I wish we had better treatments for you. We are trying so hard to develop those treatments, but we have a long way to go. As much as I want to offer you more treatment for your cancer, I am sure I would only harm you if I did. I know this news must be devastating, especially after you have traveled so far to get here." I can imagine a long period of silence as the man and his wife processed this profound information. The conversation may have proceeded as follows:

"What do you hope for now?"

"Of course, I want someone to cure my cancer, but if I am not cured, I want to live with dignity and comfort."

"What would a life with dignity and comfort look like to you now?"

"I want more than anything to go home to see my friends and family."

"I can only imagine how wonderful it would be for you to return home and how discouraging it must be to be unable to do so during the global pandemic. I heard that your home country is beautiful, especially at this time of year. What did you most enjoy doing during your spare time at home before you became ill?"

"I loved hiking in the foothills near my home year-round, especially in the snow."

"It sounds as though your illness has changed your life dramatically."

"Yes, it has changed my life, but what can I do? Sometimes we do not understand God's plan. Death is but a part of life. No one guarantees long life when we enter this world. We struggle mightily to take that first breath, never knowing when our last breath will be. Then we all choose how we live our lives and do the best we can. If this is my time, it will come much too soon, but I am grateful for the good years I have enjoyed."

"I am inspired by your courage and composure under such difficult circumstances. Caring for people like you makes my job truly meaningful. I am honored to have gotten to know you and to help care for you, even if only for a short time."

I would have then sat in silence by his side, not trying to fix the unfixable, but simply sticking with him, no matter what, just as I learned from Dr. Papa.

PRACTICE POINTS

Key Reflections

- Most people considered a diagnosis of metastatic cancer to be a death sentence until recently. However, treatment for patients with metastatic melanoma and other malignancies has improved dramatically in recent decades with the discovery of effective options, including targeted therapy and immunotherapy.

- Mentors can have a huge impact on the professional development of young physicians by demonstrating ways of connecting meaningfully with patients and their families.

- Physicians who maintain a positive "aura" and always stick by their patients no matter what build strong, trusting relationships with their patients.

- The process of making complex decisions about cancer treatment should be adapted to the unique circumstances of each patient.

- Helping patients navigate important decisions about their care, especially as their treatment options become more limited, is arguably the most important task of a good medical oncologist.

- Transitioning to a purely palliative strategy at the appropriate time is the farthest thing from "giving up."

Empathic Actions

- When doctors direct their undivided attention to patients through verbal and nonverbal means they are in essence saying, "You are all that matters to me at this moment."

- Asking patients open-ended, exploratory questions to determine what they understand about their illness, how they want to handle sensitive information, and how they want to live if treatments do not go well allows them to process complex information and offers the medical team insight regarding their level of understanding and their emotional state.

  ○ "What do you hope for now?"

  ○ "What would a life with dignity and comfort look like to you now?"

  ○ "What did you most enjoy doing during your spare time at home before you became ill?"

- Physicians should tell their patients the truth, even if the truth is scary, but should deliver the truth with compassion and empathy.

- Displaying authentic emotion in the right measure is therapeutic. Patients do not expect us to be robots. Revealing our humanity rather than always pretending everything is perfect is another way of showing that we care.

Empathic Expression

- "I admire your fighting spirit. You have traveled a long way to seek better treatments after having already fought so hard at home."

- "I respect how much you love your husband. I would like to think I would advocate for my husband if he were seriously ill as strongly as you advocate for yours."

- "I wish we had better treatments for you. We are trying so hard to develop those treatments, but we have a long way to go. As much as I want to offer you more treatment for your cancer, I am sure I would only harm you if I did."

- "I can only imagine how wonderful it would be for you to return home and how discouraging it must be to be unable to do so during the global pandemic."

- "It sounds as though your illness has changed your life dramatically."

- "I am inspired by your courage and composure under such difficult circumstances. Caring for people like you makes my job truly meaningful. I am honored to have gotten to know you and to help care for you, even if only for a short time."

7 | Tell Me Stories

Bruno P. Granwehr and Daniel E. Epner

My FATHER WAS not a sinner, far from it. He was a good man, even a great man in many ways. He filled his lungs with life like he was taking a long drag on a cigarette, and then exhaled howls of joy. He was a paradox: a black hole that gathered everyone around him into his inescapable gravitational field while emitting blindingly bright light. Yet, like all people, my father was imperfect. He could pull my mother, brother, and me into his grasp, enjoying the light and warmth, yet he sometimes unintentionally crushed those closest to him with his passion and high expectations.

The Call of Duty

My father was born on Madeira Island, Portugal and spent most of his childhood there with the exception of a few years in his father's native Switzerland. His first language was Portuguese, but he also learned Italian, English, and German while attending school. He smoked from the age of 15, eventually accumulating more than 100 pack-years, but nonetheless became a champion sprinter and swimmer during his youth. He attended medical school in Oporto, Portugal and was fascinated by so many medical disciplines that he had difficulty choosing a career path. He was initially drawn to psychiatry and the theory of mind, fascinated by the teachings of Freud and Jung. However, he became frustrated and disillusioned by the relative lack of sophistication in psychiatric diagnosis and treatment and ultimately chose anesthesia and the physiologic and technical approach to trauma and critical care. He was a clinician who viewed medicine through a scientist's lens, fascinated by the elegant design and resilience of the human body. He strove tirelessly to understand the how and why of everything and often proclaimed, "Medicine is beautiful."

In April 1974, the "Revolution of the Carnations" took place in Portugal, ending a decades' long dictatorship. My father and many others were glad to be rid of authoritarian rule, but he quickly became disenchanted with the socialist government that replaced it. He spoke out against the new government with disgust, which led others to warn him that, "There is a lamp post waiting for you." Seeing this threat as an opportunity to fulfill a dream so common to many around the world, he moved our family to the United States. He rightfully viewed the US as fertile ground for physician-scientists like himself to solve the great mysteries of the human body and its ailments, even half-jokingly suggesting he would win the Nobel Prize. My father always had an insatiable curiosity, seeking to understand the human body with the tools of science.

After our family moved to the United States in 1975, as commonly occurs with international medical graduates, my father was required to repeat residency training in anesthesia. He embraced the opportunity to take call every other day in the SICU for months on end while devoting the remaining months to other clinical duties and to intense laboratory work. Back then, work hour rules were nonexistent, and he gladly pushed himself to the limit. Being older than most of his fellow residents, my father was one of few trainees who had a family. Fortunately, my mother filled the void created by his absence the best she could, but we still missed him. My father's presence in our lives was a rare treat, like Portuguese sweet rice (arroz doce) straight from the pot on the stove on Christmas day. He maintained his frenetic pace even after transitioning to a faculty position, but he became disillusioned when departures of other faculty members cut into his research time and shattered his dreams of scientific discovery. Ever the voice of reason, my mother offered reality checks to my father's quixotic ideas, encouraging him to consider other job opportunities with more stable prospects.

As a result, he departed academia to enter private practice at Mercy Hospital in Des Moines, Iowa. Incredibly, he accelerated his work pace after making the move. Rather than focusing on a single discipline, he continued to engage in the full spectrum of anesthesia, working in critical care, but also developing expertise in cardiac, pediatric, and obstetric anesthesia. My father also enjoyed pushing boundaries to serve his patients, convincing his group and the hospital to establish a labor epidural service. He was the "go to" anesthesiologist who cardiac surgeons sought out for complicated cases, such as heart and heart-lung transplants or artificial hearts. He worked closely with a cardiac surgeon to pioneer open-heart surgery for management of acute myocardial infarction. My father had an unmatched work ethic until his retirement at the age of 65, continuing to take call for 24 or more hours at a time, which would result in work hour violations for trainees today. While my father embraced his work with all his heart, my mother, my brother, and I had many late dinners and interrupted holiday meals.

Renaissance Man

As if his work schedule were not arduous enough, my father also had an insatiable appetite for life outside of medicine. He read nonmedical journals, like *The Economist* and learned how to sail, snow ski, and play tennis at high levels as an adult. He also cultivated a lifelong love affair with soccer, playing with the "Over the Hill Gang" well into his 50s. He was well known for taking "smoking breaks" rather than water breaks on the soccer pitch and was always the last to leave the field. After smoking for 100+ pack-years, he amazingly still maintained sufficient lung function to lead his team to victory in the 400m sprint relay in the Drake University Corporate Track and Field Relays, representing his hospital. I have never seen anyone push himself as hard as my father. He was like a mountain climber who ascended all the planet's highest peaks without bottled oxygen, one after the other without rest. He was a force who could only be stopped by his own doing.

Basking in His Warmth

Occasions when I interacted meaningfully with my father during childhood were all the more memorable in light of their relative rarity. For instance, my father made optimal use of time in the car. When he drove my brother and me around, typically one-on-one, he discussed far-ranging topics, including principles of airplane flight, the history of conflict in the Middle East, and the economy of the European Union, and then quizzed us to determine our understanding. Family car rides to dinner were enjoyable, listening to his favorite music like Dave Brubeck, Miles Davis, Rosemary Clooney, Joe Jackson, and others. He also used car rides as an opportunity to discipline us. After my mother saw me do a funny walk to mock my 2nd-grade teacher behind his back, my father took me for a ride, asking, "Is that what you want to do? Would you like to be a clown for the rest of your life?" At certain times, however, he was relaxed with his discipline, "the boys are just being boys," but had high expectations that we did not wish to disappoint.

One of my most vivid memories of childhood occurred on July 4th during high school, even though I did not even experience the event first-hand. My friends and I had tickets to a concert, so we left my brother at home to fend for himself. After I returned from the concert late that night, my brother recounted the events of the evening. True to form, my father and his colleague, a cardiac surgeon, with whom he routinely played soccer, showed little interest in small fireworks like sparklers and bottle rockets but instead focused immediately on the largest, brightest, and most dangerous incendiary devices in their arsenal, all in the middle of a raging Iowa thunderstorm. They pointed them in every conceivable direction, forcing my brother to take cover under water on several occasions to avoid injury. These were two men whose hands were essential to their work, yet they could not resist the adrenaline rush of risking their careers for the excitement. That story epitomizes my father's approach to life, full of passion, intensity, and fun but occasionally reckless.

Bad News Tinged with Happiness

In late March 2018, during a visit to see my family in Iowa, my father asked me to sit while he discussed an important development. His serious tone and my mother's tears signaled bad news. I wondered, "Have my parents decided to divorce? Is my father going to move full time to our lake house in Missouri?" Instead, my father announced that he developed hemoptysis the month before and that imaging confirmed a large right upper lobe mass, sure to represent cancer. He told us, "I have lived a long life. I don't want a biopsy. I don't want treatment. I want to enjoy whatever life I have left, remain active, and spend as much time at the lake house as I can, for as long as I can." I could not comprehend how my role model, an indefatigable force, was afflicted with a disease that would soon end his life. For once in my father's life, he was not frenetically discussing a political or economic event, pitching a quality improvement project to the hospital administration, or stabilizing a crashing patient in the operating room or ICU. He was not bettering himself on the ski slopes or soccer pitch. He was fully present with my mother and me. I suggested he speak with an oncologist about options, but I respected his preference when he refused. My brother joined us at my parents' home later that evening and was as shocked by my father's news as we were. After a few minutes, the initial shock subsided and we began to reminisce about the precious times we spent together as a family, laughing and crying and cherishing an ironic celebration of life in the wake of impending death. That was arguably our best night together as a family.

True to his word, my father spent most of his remaining months at our lake home in Missouri, where he photographed nature and even did heavy work around the house and yard. Over time, he became increasingly fatigued and ultimately developed post-obstructive pneumonia. As his condition dwindled, he eventually returned to our family home in Iowa where he entered hospice and soon transitioned to inpatient hospice. When he got to the point that he could no longer take oral analgesics, the nurses decided to start an IV but had trouble finding a vein. A supervising nurse who previously worked with my father in the ER, was able to place the IV, much to our relief. While tending to him, she referred to him as "Dr. Granwehr," rather than "Joe" as a sign of respect and told my mother that she was always relieved when my father arrived in the operating room to help care for a trauma victim. She knew he would calmly "take charge" and announce that "everything was going to be alright." Through all his countless hours and nights in the ICU, in the OR, and in the ER, my father earned the unqualified respect and admiration of his peers. He died peacefully a short time later with my mother, my brother, and me at his side.

An Epiphany That Came Too Late

My father often told me, "Work is the only thing you can control," and I took his words to heart. I followed his path, but I learned some hard life lessons along the way. My children were born in Galveston, Texas, where I trained in infectious diseases and remained on faculty as my first position after completing training. When a hurricane nearly struck our home in Galveston, my wife was concerned enough to seek work closer to our families, either in Idaho or Iowa. Ultimately, we decided to move to Idaho. The move was difficult for me, with my frustrations expressed in an attempt to negotiate a position outside of Idaho, but trying to remain close to our families. Frustrated by this and with other sources of discord, my wife sought divorce, ultimately leading to my return to Texas, where I took the position at MD Anderson Cancer Center. It provided greater financial security, but I missed seeing my children and the sense of family. I rationalized my move by reminding myself that, "Work is the only thing you can control."

My son was just four and my daughter just two when my wife and I divorced in 2007. Over time, my sense of duty and devotion turned into a sense of loneliness and loss as I missed spending time with my family. I felt as though my father had sold me a false promise. Yes, we have little control over many forces in our lives, but we have control over our intentions. I realized that I may not be able to attend every birthday party and holiday dinner, but I could always make my family my highest priority rather than worshiping the golden idol of work. I spent time with my children when they stayed with me every summer, spring break, and the holidays, as well as spending weekends in Idaho, but I missed birthdays, including those of my parents and brother, and realized I was too often distracted by work. As noted by Harold Kushner, "No one ever said on their death bed, 'I wish I'd spent more time at the office.'" This advice is as valuable as it is cliché. Unfortunately, this epiphany came after too many missed birthdays and holiday celebrations.

Expressions to Live By

One of my father's favorite expressions was "Medicine is beautiful." I know he loved practicing medicine and could not imagine another career path, but I have always wondered what he meant by "beautiful." Perhaps he was referring to how beautifully integrated biological systems are within the human body or to the beauty of deciphering those systems. He also found beauty in holding a young child's hand to soothe his fears before surgery. Based on his faith in the science of medicine, he was an early advocate for statins for his known heart disease, and underwent angioplasty on four occasions during his life, starting in his early 40s. Faced with a grave illness at the end of his life, however, he refused the full spectrum of diagnostic and therapeutic approaches of modern medicine. I will never know for sure what he meant by "Medicine is beautiful," but after practicing medicine for several years, I now have my own ideas.

One of my father's favorite expressions was "Tell me stories," often spoken with a cigarette dangling from his lips. He probably started using that expression during his youth on Madeira Island, famous in Portugal as "Gossip Central," the place where neighborhood gossip achieved status as high art form. When I was growing up, the first thing my father said upon arriving home from work was "Tell me stories" to learn about my day at school. He also loved to swap stories with friends and colleagues and often laughed infectiously when telling or receiving amusing tales. He seemed to understand that stories lie at the intersection of science and humanity, at a place where quantifiable data points merge with the human experience of illness. I now think when my father said, "Medicine is beautiful" he meant that caring for his most vulnerable patients with great humanity was a beautiful experience. I take the same stance with my patients. As a specialist in infectious diseases, I formulate differential diagnoses primarily by an extensive history combined with review of culture and laboratory results, imaging, and physical exam findings. However, I need to connect with my patients on a human level to develop a diagnostic and treatment plan that best suits their unique circumstances and perspectives.

A Bigger Hug

Like my father, I have always encouraged my son and daughter to tell me stories, although without a cigarette dangling from my lips. My children, like all people, have a fundamental need to be heard. By sharing stories, my children test ideas, share burdens, and solidify their identities, so listening to them is one of the most powerful ways to maintain and build our connection. Unlike my father's in-depth queries, I set no particular agenda when I see my kids. I try to resist the temptation to bombard them with unsolicited advice but am happy to impart wisdom whenever they want. Early on, I was tempted to indulge them excessively out of a sense of guilt, but over time I have learned to strike a balance between unconditional love and a healthy dose of structure and discipline. The thing I love the most about being with them is just being with them.

Last year, during my son's junior year of high school, I urged him to apply to any college he wanted, anywhere in the country. However, he insisted on applying to schools in Houston so he could live close to me, and this fall, he will enroll at the University of Houston. My daughter is a rising high school junior who has also decided to move to Houston to finish her last two years of high school. I have made many mistakes in my life, but I must have done something right. My father was an imperfect man, exhibiting such a high intensity and standard for himself that he imposed on others, excessive at times, prioritizing work over all else. Work-life balance was not in his vocabulary until he retired, finally realizing the enjoyment in simple labor around the house, reading, and family events. He was a man who ultimately taught me to embrace life as a gift to be treasured and lived to its fullest. Our family and friends provide the human connections that make us whole, the connections that provide us the energy, compassion, and empathy to treat our patients as whole human beings…to hear stories.

PRACTICE POINTS

Key Reflections

- Medicine is a beautiful profession, where science meets humanity.

- Striking a balance between work and other priorities, particularly family, allows most clinicians to maintain the highest level of passion, energy, and effectiveness as they care for patients.

- Clinicians should also advise their patients to maintain work-life balance in order to maintain their physical and emotional health.

- All people have a fundamental need to be heard. Receiving patients' stories is the key to understanding their perspectives and adapting to their needs and priorities.

- Some patients subscribe to the "less is more" philosophy, knowing some of the complications of medical interventions, performing their own risk-benefit analysis, and opting for a less aggressive, more humanistic approach.

- Sometimes even the simplest gestures, like finding out whether a patient prefers to be called by first or last name, communicate respect and strengthen connection.

Empathic Actions

- Spending time with patients, colleagues, friends, and family, sometimes with no particular agenda, is a powerful way of saying "I care."

- People often feel as though they have little control over many forces in their lives, but they still retain control over their intentions.

Empathic Expression

- Tell me stories.

- I know we can always count on you. You are our "go to" doctor. When you come around, I know everything is going to be alright.

8 | Paying It Forward

Linda C. Epner and Daniel E. Epner

A Grandmother's Challenge

I was born in the small city of Hsinchu, Taiwan, where we lived with my paternal grandparents during the two years that my father worked on his doctorate at Vanderbilt. My father's family was of very modest means, since my grandfather was a police officer during the Japanese occupation of Taiwan, and my grandmother Mae was a homemaker with 11 children, of whom my father was the 10th. My grandmother had a major impact on my life, especially with regard to my work as a physician. I followed her around all day as a toddler, accompanying her as she shopped in open-air markets, performed her daily chores, and cooked. She treated me like a tiny person, almost like an adult, but she also sternly set limits with me when necessary. Though she never had formal education, Grandmother Mae had a sharp mind and an otherworldly wisdom. She could instantly calculate the total cost of her groceries in her head without the aid of an abacus, and she could judge a person's character by keenly observing their body language and demeanor. She was a woman of few words and deep thoughts who always remained composed despite their financial hardships and the stress of raising such a large family. When she spoke, her words invariably carried love, wisdom, and encouragement. What she lacked in material possessions she more than made up for with love.

When my father was nearly done with his doctorate, he felt secure enough in his future to bring us to America to join him in his tiny apartment. I sometimes joke with my two young adult daughters that I swam all the way from Taiwan to the United States at age three with a winter melon strapped to my back for floatation, which is the equivalent to a midwesterner claiming to have walked to and from school every day barefoot in the snow, uphill both ways. However, we actually traveled by commercial airline. My entire extended family saw us off at the airport because they understood the profound significance of our journey. They knew we would visit in the future but that we would never again live in Taiwan. In fact, it took my parents a decade before they saved enough money to fly back. Occasionally when I look through old family albums, I come across the black and white photo of my sister, my mother, and me posing at my paternal grandparents' house on the morning of our departure to America. My mother smiled proudly wearing a pearl necklace, shiny black high-heeled shoes, and a form-fitting dress and matching jacket that appeared traditionally Chinese yet modern and fashionable at the same time. I cannot imagine how my mother tolerated wearing that dress during the 24-hour journey to America accompanied by two toddlers. She clearly understood the enormity of leaving her extensive support system behind in Taiwan in search of a better life in America, so she dressed to honor the occasion.

Many years later, after I entered medical school, I traveled back to Taiwan to see my Grandmother Mae for what proved to be the last time. While there, she told me the story of when my father broke his arm as a little boy over 80 years ago, but no doctor was available in Hsinchu to fix it. They heard that a doctor lived in the adjacent town so they walked for many hours to seek help, having no other means of transportation. My grandfather literally carried my father in his arms the whole way to ease my father's tremendous pain. When they reached the doctor, they told him with great trepidation that they had no money to pay him, expecting him to turn them away. However, he instead silently swiveled around in his chair, examined my father's arm, and fixed it without fanfare. He did not even look up into their eyes, since he must have known how ashamed they were to be unable to pay him. The kind doctor only suggested that they bring him a small token of appreciation later if they were able. A year later, my grandparents carried an adult chicken to him that they had lovingly raised since the time of my father's injury. A chicken may not sound like much by today's standards, but in Taiwan during the late 1930s, it was very valuable. Thinking that my grandmother had finished telling the story, I started to say how impressed I was by the doctor's altruism and by my grandparents' expression of appreciation. However, she stopped me to say that she had not yet gotten to the most important part. She explained that they did not actually pay their debt to the kind doctor with the chicken, no matter how valuable it was at the time. The chicken was a mere symbol. Instead, she told me that it was now my destiny to pay back society for the doctor's kindness through my future service as a doctor. I should care for everyone regardless of his or her ability to pay. I tell this story because it had an indelible impact on me, having come from a woman whom I idealized as much as anyone in the world. That story became my professional and personal North Star.

When I finished my residency training, I considered various practice scenarios and even worked for a short time at an HMO and subsequently in private practice. However, I soon gravitated to positions that gave me the opportunity to care for underserved patients from minority and indigent communities, much like the one where my father grew up. The first such position I held was at a Baltimore inner-city clinic affiliated with the Wilmer Eye Institute at Johns Hopkins, where I held a faculty position during my husband's fellowship training. The more I settled into these jobs, the more natural they felt to me. Over the past 26 years, I have practiced ophthalmology in an academic setting, serving underserved communities in a county safety-net clinic and teaching ophthalmology residents small incision cataract surgery in the operating rooms at a Veterans Administration Medical Center. Ophthalmology is one of the most lucrative medical specialties, so working in the public sector with a largely indigent population for relatively little money as I have done is extraordinarily unusual. Sometimes I think about moving to private practice, but then I remember my Grandmother Mae's challenge for me and I continue to follow my true calling.

Emulating the Taiwanese Country Doctor

I can best explain my philosophy of patient care with an example from my community safety-net clinic. My templates often have more than 35 patients per day, and patients can wait up to several months to see me. So, nearly all of my patients show up every day, rain or shine, from near and far, regardless of the circumstances. For example, Houston experiences severe flooding once or twice nearly every year, but my patients nonetheless find their way to clinic. Many of my patients have young children, but they do not have the luxury to hire babysitters when they go to the doctor, so they often bring their children to appointments with me. I often find myself examining a mom while surrounded by her toddlers as they breathe on my elbows and peer curiously at the slit lamp. This arrangement would never fly in a private office, but in our community health clinics, it is often unavoidable.

One day when patients packed into the waiting room, the dilation room, and retina scan room as usual, I heard a commotion in the hallway as I was examining a patient. When I peeked out to see what was going on, I noticed a young mother struggling with her two rambunctious boys, both of whom were tugging at leashes attached to harnesses around their chests. The leashes were the kind that parents occasionally use at large amusement parks to keep their 2- to 3-year-old children from wandering off into the crowd. However, these boys were at least 4 and 6 years old, and were big for their age, so the woman was struggling as if she were trying to corral two wild horses. She was frazzled and desperate. As I gazed upon this chaotic scene playing out in the waiting room, I contemplated whether I should see her then or ask my staff to reschedule her on a day when she could come alone. I have to admit I was sorely tempted to reschedule her. Not only was it almost impossible to examine her in the midst of such chaos, but I also had an obligation to my other patients, who stared angrily at the boys with the loud music blaring from their electronic tablets. After a few seconds, I went with my gut instinct and decided to see her. I am a mother of two children, albeit less energetic ones, but being a mother allowed me to realize that no woman on earth would choose to bring her two children to a doctor's appointment if she could possibly avoid it. She must have been under extreme duress and desperate to see me if she was willing to endure the angry glares of all the other patients. I soon learned that this 30-year-old woman had experienced several types of severe trauma during her childhood and adolescence, including sexual trauma, mental illness, and abuse at the hands of multiple family members, including her husband, who was in jail. In addition, her sons had attention deficit disorder, which seemed obvious, so she could not find anyone, including her own mother, willing to look after them for a few hours. She presented to my office because she was having splitting headaches for months, and her primary care doctor thought she needed glasses. Her primary care physician (PCP) also referred her to a neurologist, but that appointment was several months in the future, and she could no longer endure the severe headaches.

As soon as I started to take her history, even before examining her, I could tell her headaches were not due to lack of glasses.

She looked exhausted and anxious and had pressured speech but was nonetheless of sound mind. She wore a backpack stuffed with food, juice boxes, and clothing and repeatedly yelled at her boys to sit still and be quiet. She explained that her vision came in and out and that she had weird areas where she could not see anything. No one who had examined her could make a diagnosis, so they urged her to get plenty of sleep, take Tylenol as needed, and wait for the neurology appointment. Fortunately, the nursing staff was willing to entertain the boys with tongue depressors and inflated latex gloves long enough for me to look at her eyes, which revealed severe bilateral papilledema, strongly suggesting idiopathic intracranial hypertension. In retrospect, she fit the classic demographic as a young, obese woman. Nonetheless, no one had made the diagnosis, which is relatively rare and would have remained a mystery for at least several more months if I had not agreed to see her.

My next step was to confirm the diagnosis with neuroimaging to rule out a brain tumor or other focal lesion and to perform lumbar puncture, both of which were beyond the capabilities of my clinic. I knew I would need to convince her to go to the county hospital emergency room immediately for evaluation, which would be no small task under the circumstances.

I have never had the privilege of formal communication skills training, since such training did not exist when I was in medical school and residency. We just learned by watching faculty mentors and repeating the phrases we thought sounded good without understanding why they may actually be effective under various circumstances. I therefore did not possess an extensive repertoire of empathic phrases. Still, I knew I would need to make every effort to impress upon her the severity of her condition by using whatever skills I have developed by practicing medicine for many years. My first strategy was to be completely transparent and honest. I started by saying:

"I realize you just met me, so you have no reason to trust me. The easiest thing for me would be to tell you to wait for the neurology appointment and get some more sleep, or try new glasses. However, doing those things will not relieve your headaches. I know you need more tests that I cannot do here. I want you to go to the county hospital to get those tests, even though I realize doing so will be very difficult for you. I will call my colleagues there to speed things up, but you will still probably have to wait many hours in the emergency room."

I listened quietly for a few minutes as she told me a little more about her life's hardships and then said, "Sounds rough. You're doing the best you can." I then described her medical condition in plain language:

"The nerves that connect your eyes to your brain are swollen, probably because the pressure in your head is elevated, which is why you have such bad headaches. This is an emergency. I really want you to go to the emergency room to get those tests. I wish I could do them for you here."

She first looked at me with skepticism, but after looking me in the eyes, she must have concluded I was telling the truth, because she went to the emergency room where tests confirmed the diagnosis. I believe I gained her trust by listening to her describe hardships in her life during the visit and by later explaining her presumed diagnosis in plain language. She must have also appreciated the fact that I agreed to see her as an overbook appointment with her rambunctious boys. In other words, I earned her trust quickly by imagining how difficult her life must be and by taking empathic action. I am sure I spoke empathically, but my actions were more empathic than my words.

Mental Health Issues in Ophthalmology Clinic

Asking people about their lives helps me decide what direction to go with the exam and how best to help them. My patients are under tremendous stress, like most people, but probably to a greater degree due to financial limitations and mental illness. The majority of my patients see me to evaluate problems that their referring doctors think are ophthalmic but ultimately prove not to be. I have to size up the situation very quickly and triage patients, because my templates are so full every day. For instance, I see many patients to evaluate headaches or uncontrollable blinking. Many of my patients are children who are not doing well in school, ostensibly because they cannot see the chalkboard or they appear unable to read. Pediatricians often refer children who they think need glasses, but in most cases, they have no refractive error.

For instance, I recently saw a little girl with her mother because she was constantly blinking, rubbing her eyes, and not paying attention in school, so her schoolwork was suffering. Her teacher was concerned and told her mom to make an appointment with her pediatrician, who promptly referred her to me. She was a very sad-looking, anxious child whose visual acuity was 20/20, so she clearly did not need glasses. I did note, however, that all her eyelashes were either missing or broken, so I quickly realized she was pulling her eyelashes out one by one, perhaps unconsciously, a condition known as trichotillomania. I asked her how she was doing in her classes, whether she felt nervous at school, or whether other kids were bullying her. As I delved into her story, I realized that her school environment was just fine but that she was having trouble concentrating because she missed her father. The little girl's mother had recently thrown her father out of the house for a malfeasance that she did not describe in any detail. As a result, the girl had not seen her father for a while and was afraid she may never see him again. She was sleeping poorly and was nervously pulling out her eyelashes, which caused dust and debris to accumulate in her eyes. As a result, she was constantly rubbing them and creating micro-corneal abrasions: a vicious cycle that prevented her from concentrating on her schoolwork.

This little girl's ophthalmic issues were attributable to fear and sadness. In the process of trying to reduce stress in her life by parting ways with the girl's father, her mother had paradoxically increased her stress. After I brought this reality to light, the girl's mother realized that her daughter still loved her father even though he acted like a jerk at times, and she was able to reassure her that she would still get to see him periodically in a supervised environment. I then gave her lubricating drops, asked her to use them whenever she felt nervous, and reassured her she would be much better in no time. When she returned several months later, she had seen her father several times without incident and all of her eyelashes had grown back.

This little girl with no eyelashes epitomizes my patients, many of whom have psychiatric and psychosocial challenges that profoundly inhibit their ability to function in society. I often sit in my examining room and listen to sounds emanating from the waiting area to pick up all sorts of issues, including the rapid speech of manic patients, fear in the voice of anxious patients, or repetitive handwashing of obsessive-compulsive patients. Schizophrenics display the customary vacant stares or bizarre speech patterns and appearance. When I trained in ophthalmology, I did not realize that I would have to serve a dual role as therapist.

To compound the complexity of my work, my clinic is located in a huge, ethnically diverse metropolitan area in southeast Texas, so I see many immigrants who have traveled far to seek a safer or better life, just as my family did over 50 years ago. My waiting room looks like the United Nations, with many patients from central and South America, Africa, Asia, Eastern Europe, and even exotic locales like Nepal. Regardless of the political debates raging about immigration, I feel an obligation to care for my patients to the best of my ability regardless of their nationality. Most of the children I see do not have dyslexia or refractive errors or other unusual ophthalmic issues; they are just experiencing posttraumatic stress disorder related to their arduous journey to the United States or other stressors that are common to people everywhere. Many of my patients have never had access to medical care, so they walk around for decades effectively blind and are profoundly grateful when they finally get their first pair of glasses.

An Important Role Model

Much of the work of ophthalmologists takes place in operating rooms, so we rarely if ever receive formal training that focuses on relational or psychosocial aspects of medical practice. In addition, I rarely get to see other ophthalmologists interact with patients. Nonetheless, one of my mentors, Morton Goldberg, former director of the Wilmer Eye Institute at Johns Hopkins, has had a profound impact on the way I care for my patients.

I first met Dr. Goldberg shortly after my husband and I moved to Baltimore for his oncology fellowship. We knew that we would likely live in Baltimore for only three years before returning to Texas to be near family after my husband finished his training, but I wanted to pursue the best career opportunities I could while I was there. I had already secured a part-time position in private practice before arriving in Baltimore, but I sought an additional position at the Wilmer that would fulfill my desire to keep my hand in academia and to serve the underserved community. When I contacted Dr. Goldberg, he was not recruiting new faculty, but he nonetheless agreed to interview me. That was the first time I witnessed Dr. Goldberg's empathy, because he must have known how vulnerable I felt in a new city. I think many academic leaders of his stature would have summarily dismissed me or approached our meeting with arrogance, but Dr. Goldberg instead listened to me carefully and treated me with the same respect as he showed his own faculty members and other prominent academic leaders. He asked me what I thought I could offer to his department, and I told him I could teach his residents small incision cataract surgery using phacoemulsification, which at the time was still quite novel. He also invited me to attend all Johns Hopkins Ophthalmology

Grand Rounds as a way of integrating me into the ophthalmology community in Baltimore.

Then, one day a few months later, he requested that I meet him in his office again. He explained that he had heard from other ophthalmologists in the community that I had an excellent reputation as a surgeon. After much reflection, he offered me a position on his faculty to do exactly what I had proposed during our first meeting, and I agreed to his offer with just a handshake. We never had a contract, and we never needed one, because both of us were true to our words. He even reimbursed my other practice for expenses they incurred because of the arrangement, creating a win-win situation for everyone.

This story illustrates how Dr. Goldberg modeled empathy toward colleagues in ways that I now apply toward my patients. He knew that trust, respect, and presence create the foundation of our strongest relationships with colleagues and patients. On a very practical level, he wanted to ensure his residents were getting a good educational experience, and he knew my role was important in helping him achieve that goal. Whenever he saw me at Grand rounds, he would always pull me aside to ask me how the residents were doing, whether any were particularly outstanding or if any were struggling. He truly wanted honest feedback from anyone regardless of academic rank. He also regularly expressed his appreciation for my hard work teaching the residents and for taking a job that, frankly, many other faculty members found stressful.

However, to Dr. Goldberg, I was much more than just a junior faculty member who supervised his residents in the operating room a few days a week. After my husband and I had our first daughter, Margeaux, near the end of our time in Baltimore when I was still on maternity leave, Dr. Goldberg welcomed me to take Margeaux with me in a stroller to attend Grand Rounds. In fact, Dr. Goldberg even encouraged me to return to the OR a few more times before we left to return to Texas, "to be fair to the residents I had not yet taught," even though doing so meant Margeaux would have to wait in a stroller in the surgical lounge under my husband's watchful eye. Perhaps I subconsciously remembered these gracious gestures when I agreed to see the overwhelmed woman with idiopathic intracranial hypertension in my clinic that day instead of turning her away.

Even now in his 80s Dr. Goldberg still takes the time to remember the names and personal details of every faculty member who has ever worked in his department, not to mention their spouses and children. I channel Dr. Goldberg now when I take a few minutes to ask residents about their families and lives outside work before we scrub into the OR every Monday morning. I did not need formal communication skills training to learn that listening to people carefully and treating them with respect and humanity is a powerful form of empathy, because it gives me a glimpse into their personal lives and thereby helps me understand their experiences. I learned that by watching Dr. Goldberg, who was the most powerful academic ophthalmologist at one of the world's most famous medical institutions, but who nonetheless displayed the generous heart of a country doctor.

Enduring Lessons

As I drive to work each day, my mind often returns to the story my grandmother Mae told me about the country doctor in Taiwan who fixed my father's broken arm over 80 years ago, and my grandmother's directive for me to pay his good deed forward. When I think about how I treat my patients and colleagues, I often ask myself, "What would Dr. Goldberg do in this situation?" Then I think about that old black and white photo of my mother, my sister, and me on the day of our journey to America so many years ago. The elegant dress she wore that day appears dark gray in the photo, but I know exactly what hue it was, because I wore it at my medical school graduation more than 20 years later. It was crimson, like blood. To my mother, that dress symbolized many things. It symbolized the good luck and prosperity we so desperately needed at such a momentous time in our lives. The dress also symbolized the melding of old and new cultures, ancient Chinese ideals merging with the gleaming, brand new world of opportunity in America. Finally, my mother's dress symbolized the power of a family's love to bind one generation to the next ad infinitum. That dress still hangs in a place of honor in my closet, waiting for one of my daughters to wear it at some grand occasion as a reminder of Grandmother Mae's simple wish to pay it forward.

PRACTICE POINTS

Key Reflections

- Family members can be guiding lights that help physicians navigate their career paths and determine their destinies.

- The immigrant experience often creates challenges and hardships that motivate physicians to give back to those in society who are less fortunate than they are.

- Physicians who have not had the benefit of formal communication skills training during their careers can nonetheless acquire key skills by emulating professional mentors who model those skills in their interactions with patients and colleagues.

- When physicians listen to patients and colleagues carefully and treat them with respect and humanity, they get a glimpse into their personal lives and thereby gain a better understanding of their experiences.

Empathic Actions

- Adapting to a patient's needs, such as by agreeing to overbook a desperate patient under trying circumstances, is one way of demonstrating a physician's deep empathy.

- The most empathic physicians are those who not only respond to emotions with empathy, but also constantly strive to improve their technical skills and knowledge to be poised to make sound, and at times highly insightful, decisions on behalf of their patients.

- One of the most empathic actions a physician can perform is devoting the time and effort needed to establish an unusual diagnosis that has evaded other clinicians.

- A career devoted to serving the underserved can be as gratifying as or more gratifying than a financially lucrative one.

- Physicians build trust when they give their patients at least a few minutes to describe their lives, especially hardships in their lives.

- Explaining complex medical concepts in plain language that patients can understand involves imagining what the patient is thinking and feeling, which is the essence of empathy.

Empathic Expression

- "I realize you just met me, so you have no reason to trust me. The easiest thing for me would be to tell you to wait for the neurology appointment and get some more sleep, or try new glasses. However, doing those things will not relieve your headaches."

- "I know you need more tests that I cannot do here. I want you to go to the county hospital to get those tests, even though I realize doing so will be very difficult for you. I will call my colleagues there to speed things up, but you will still probably have to wait many hours in the emergency room."

- "Sounds rough. You're doing the best you can."

- "I wish I had the equipment here in my office to do the tests required to diagnose your problem, but I am afraid I need to refer you to the emergency center to do them."

9 | The Last Vestige

 of Control

Kevin Madden and Laura Meyer

ONE OF MY most vivid memories of being hospitalized as a child was awakening in the middle of the night with my bed sheets soaked in blood. I was alone, since parents were not allowed to sleep in the hospital back then. I walked down the hall to find someone to help, noticed two doctors sitting in a workroom scribbling on charts, and stood in the doorway frozen in silence until they noticed me, cleaned me up, and gave me a fresh gown. The blood was just a blown IV, but it looked like death to a terrified 7-year-old boy. The next evening, when my parents left to go home after visiting hours were over, I told them, "I won't see you tomorrow." When they asked why, I said, "I am going to die tonight."

A Rare Illness

Our family grew up on a river in New Jersey, so we spent countless hours playing in and around the water. I was usually exhilarated and energized by excursions on our boat, but the summer when I was seven I remember feeling oppressive fatigue and excruciating joint pains. I think I slept for 15 or 16 hours a day. When my symptoms persisted for several days, my parents sought help from the pediatrician in our small town, but he had no idea what was wrong with me. Back in those days, people stayed in the hospital until their doctors established a diagnosis, so I was hospitalized for over four months, initially in my hometown and later in a major medical center in New York City. My doctors eventually diagnosed Lyme disease, which had just been described at the time. I was one of the first pediatric cases.

I was eventually cured with antibiotics, but not before experiencing considerable trauma. At one point my doctors were concerned that I had developed Bell's palsy, so they did a lumbar puncture. At that time, lumbar punctures and other procedures were done very differently as compared to now. These days, one or more parent is allowed in the room, and kids get full conscious sedation. Back then, my mom was forced to wait outside while a medical assistant held me in a fetal position wide awake as the doctor injected lidocaine at the puncture site. Everything around me—the air, the fluorescent lights, and the steel table — was cold. Lumbar punctures remain common in pediatrics practice to rule out meningitis in febrile kids, but throughout my pediatrics training, I never felt comfortable doing one. I always imagined myself on the table with the needle in my back.

The Private Worlds of Dying Children

Another very traumatic memory I have from my hospitalization was when my roommate, who was a burn victim, woke up in the middle of the night screaming hysterically. Several people rushed into our room and whisked him away, after which we never saw him again. I remember describing the episode to the other kids in the playroom the next day, but no one said much. It must be very hard for kids to fully understand what's going on, so they make sense of events around them the best they can.

Sick kids who face the real prospect of death often develop a distorted picture of life, sort of half fantasy and half concrete. None of the doctors, nurses, or other staff ever talked to us about the trauma of seeing somebody carted away. We all just concluded he died, which seemed logical considering how gravely ill he and most of us were. Myra Bluebond-Langner described this informal, underground communication network among hospitalized kids in her book *The Private Worlds of Dying Children*. Whether they're dying or not, hospitalized kids occupy a private world that adults cannot access or understand. I think clinicians access that world a little bit better now than they did 40 years ago when I was hospitalized, since now we have child life specialists, child psychologists, social workers, chaplains, art therapists, and other interventions. I see my job in palliative/supportive care as coordinating with all these different disciplines to assemble the many puzzle pieces of a child's life into a coherent picture. In the end, I was cured of Lyme disease, but the longer I was hospitalized before the doctors made the diagnosis, the more I became convinced I was dying. Those visceral memories of fear, isolation, and helplessness now guide my clinical practice profoundly.

We Think He Will Talk to You

I recently cared for a boy who, like me, was in the hospital for months. He had already been hospitalized for about three months by the time his oncologist asked us to help manage his symptoms and address goals of care. Like so many of the kids admitted to our cancer center, he was suffering from the effects of progressive, incurable malignancy. He was 11, but he looked more like seven or eight. He was very cachectic and debilitated and could barely walk after being mostly bed-bound for months. His parents, like many parents of children who have serious illnesses, operated under the principle that they would do everything possible to save their child's life. It may be hard for others to understand, but parents make a type of Faustian bargain throughout their child's treatment. In the beginning, they are more than willing to sacrifice their child's quality of life in hopes of achieving cure. They consent to chemotherapy even though it causes fatigue, nausea, social isolation from peers at school, and many other side effects. As the illness progresses and the child's condition worsens, the stakes become higher and parents become ever more willing to concede quality of life to seek an increasingly elusive cure. This transition occurs gradually, so parents lose perspective and are willing to do things that they may not have otherwise chosen in the past. There's a tendency in medicine to judge parents who act like this by identifying them as being "in denial." However, I don't think we understand what it's like to have a child who faces the real prospect of death, the stark reality that at some point in the near future they will no longer be able to laugh with the child, or simply watch him breathe. Parents view their primary role as protector, so they feel that they have not fulfilled that duty if their child dies, even if that belief seems irrational to others.

After I had seen this boy for a few days, his parents started to ask me to speak in the hallway outside his room, where they would say, "He's very anxious and he's crying. He is telling us that he is afraid of dying and is afraid of getting sicker. We think he will talk to you." Their request for me to speak frankly with their son about death was unusual, since I get the opposite request from most parents, who attempt to shield their children from the truth. The hard part is usually reassuring the parents that we're just going to talk about the child's understanding of what they know, and respect their boundaries. But in this case, I had full permission to talk to him about anything.

Adapting to the Child's Needs

Whenever I talk to a child about death and dying, I first make sure they know that our time together is for their benefit rather than mine. Sometimes I have to be direct and work quickly when I know the child is rapidly approaching death. Under those circumstances, I operate under the premise that many others have not been honest, which is why they are asking me to help out at the very end of the child's life. Kids do not want to think that others can read them so easily, so I normalize the situation: "I've worked with a lot of kids who are in your situation, and they're often really scared if people haven't been honest with them or if they feel like people have kept information from them. Do you feel that way or have you ever felt that way?" Externalizing the conversation to other kids, and then asking them if they identify with those other kids, rather than directly asking, "Are you scared?" makes the conversation so much safer. Kids rarely want to answer a direct question about fear or anxiety, especially soon after meeting someone. After I try to normalize what is admittedly a very abnormal situation, I cede control of the conversation to the child. I often say something like, "This is your opportunity to talk, but only if you want to. Do you want to tell me more? If you don't, that's okay. I don't need you to. But here's your opportunity to ask the questions that you probably are thinking about or want to know the answers to." When I approach sensitive conversations with children, I neither shield them from the truth nor impose it upon them, but rather adapt to each kid's unique needs.

In the case of my 11-year-old patient, he was gravely ill but not imminently dying, so I had some time to get to know him rather than taking a very direct approach. I wanted to fulfill his parents' desire for me to learn more about the boy's fear of death and help him cope, but I tried not to control the agenda when we met. I did not want to feel like I was trying to check a box on my to-do list. My goal was to give him total control over the relationship in the beginning in hopes of gaining his trust. I said, in essence, "I'm on your turf. This is your home, and I am a guest in it. I don't want to spend any more time here than you find valuable. I don't want to waste your time." This approach gave him a tiny measure of control over his life by letting him make a decision, even a seemingly small one. Kids who are hospitalized for a long time are violated in so many different ways, and they lose control over just about every aspect of their lives. When kids withhold access to their private world they exert what is arguably their last vestige of control, which is a normal and healthy way of preserving whatever identity and dignity they still possess.

Day after day, I entered his room, sat beside him, and asked open-ended and non-medical questions to encourage him to express himself. For instance, I sometimes asked him about one of his favorite TV programs or a sporting event. After a few weeks, I began to notice that his parents would quietly leave the room after a few minutes while we were engrossed in conversation, leaving just me and the boy. I knew his parents wanted me to speak to him about his fears of death, so I tried to gently probe in many different ways by asking him how he was feeling. However, I have learned that children only trust a few people enough to allow them access to their inner thoughts, and sometimes I am not one of those people. As the days passed, I continued to tread lightly, looking at pictures on his phone and discussing his interests. The last thing I wanted was for him to feel as though I was trying to extract medical data from him or unload unwanted information on him. I then tried to normalize his situation by comparing his experiences to those of other children with similar illnesses. I told him, "You know, other kids who are in the hospital for a long time often wonder if they're getting sicker or whether they might die. Do you ever wonder that?" I encouraged him to share his fears with me in many different ways, but he would always respond, "No, I'm okay. I'm okay." Afterward, his parents would catch me in the hallway very eager to hear what he told me, and each day, I repeated, "Nothing. He doesn't tell me much of anything. I keep asking him in many different ways, but he doesn't want to tell me anything, and I think that's okay. I'm not going to push him."

There's something magical about how kids live in the moment and see the world in a very visceral and vibrant way. I am forever inspired and humbled working with seriously ill children. I often find myself thinking, "These kids—yes they hide a lot of stuff, but in the end they are still much more resilient than adult patients with similar illnesses."

I learned from one of my mentors that I should never harass kids with kindness in an attempt to get information, because they can see right through it. Kids do not want to feel as if they are being deceived or manipulated. They probably think, "That's great. That's what you want and what you get out of it, but what about me?" Maybe a child does not want to talk about a particular topic, or maybe he just does not want to talk to me. I resisted the temptation to reach for something that wasn't there, so we never talked about death and other deep topics. Instead of seeing my visits as opportunities to accomplish some larger goal, I realized at some point that the most I could do was to meet him where he was every day. I was still his doctor, and I addressed his medical needs, but our relationship turned into more of a friendship. He just needed to feel like a normal kid and forget about his circumstances for at least a few minutes every day.

I eventually stumbled upon reading books to him. Most of the time he would fall asleep within five minutes of me reading and I would just keep reading for a while. For the last two weeks of his life, about the only thing I did was read a book aloud to him for 20 or 30 minutes every day. He was very intelligent, so he probably knew at some level that he was dying. I also believe that he had some conception that death could happen to him, but we never talked about it.

Gratitude

After a few weeks, he went to the ICU to receive high flow oxygen to maintain normal saturations, but he did not require other intensive interventions. By that time, his oncologists had acknowledged that they could no longer safely treat his malignancy, which was completely out of control and making him feel sicker. This occurred during the COVID-19 pandemic, so his parents and two brothers were not allowed to visit. His brothers were several years older and were working in other cities, but they relocated to Houston to be near him during his hospitalization. Of course, everyone in the hospital was frustrated and saddened by the restrictive visitation policies during the pandemic, but his brothers were particularly angry and did not hesitate to voice their feelings. This was one circumstance when the pandemic, despite all its brutality, ironically offered a silver lining, because it opened up another strategy for me to speak about how to best take care of this young boy. I was never able to speak explicitly with the boy about his fears, as his parents wanted me to. However, when his family voiced their understandable frustration about not being able to see him at such a delicate time, I finally said, "If you want to be able to see him, we need to get him out of the hospital, and I worry that there is a very narrow window in which to do so." I felt at that moment that his brothers needed my most direct, unambiguous message to help them crystallize their thoughts. A window of opportunity opened when we were able to wean his oxygen to levels that could be supported at home. Even then, I did not frame the decision to go home with hospice as a one-way ticket. Instead, I asked, "Why don't you go home for just a few days and see what happens?" This question at least left open the hypothetical possibility that he could return if he or his family wanted. In essence, my question offered them an insurance policy or a security blanket, like "The door is always open." Fortunately, he died peacefully at home a few days later.

Caring for this boy and many other children like him has changed my perspective, which seems only natural considering I have three children, ages, 4, 5, and 12. I often find myself looking at my kids for just a fraction of a second longer to stop and just *be* with them in that moment more deliberately than I once did. Then the epiphany follows: "Wow! I take all of this for granted most of the time, but there are many parents who will never see the world in the same way again because their child died today. I am incredibly lucky. I can't imagine what it would be like to be a parent of a seriously ill child." I had a similar epiphany after my wife experienced cardiac arrest and nearly died in the hospital due to a medication error shortly after the birth of our 12-year-old son. During the agonizing minutes before I found out she was ok, I seriously contemplated the terrifying prospect of raising my newborn son as a single parent. These reflections, just imaging the unthinkable, serve as raw material for my empathic practice.

A New Perspective

For a while after this young boy died, I thought, "Did I do the right thing? Could I have kept trying to get him to open up to me in other ways? Should I have been more direct in an effort to get him home sooner?" I was not sure how much I had helped him and his family by doing almost nothing other than reading to him every day. Then I attended his funeral.

His funeral was unlike any I had attended before. The boy's favorite place in the world during his illness was his bed at home. So, his family re-created his bedroom for the funeral by bringing in his nightstand, bookcase, and bed, where he lay in peaceful repose. They even brought his beloved dog, who always slept at the foot of the bed and sat faithfully in that spot throughout the funeral. In addition to placing the boy's body in his bed during the funeral rather than in a casket, his family also created an elaborate 35-minute video tribute to honor his life. The video gave mourners a sense of how full his life was, even during his prolonged cancer ordeal. As I watched the video, one of the first thoughts that entered my mind was, "When did this kid ever get chemotherapy, between countless trips to exotic and luxurious destinations?" His parents must have known he was likely to die of his illness, because they made every effort imaginable to ensure he lived life to the fullest, even between cycles of chemotherapy, and to document many of those experiences. It was almost as if they were creating their own legacy memorial in real-time. He literally traveled around the world during the months before his final hospitalization. The second thought that entered my mind was, "As much as I thought I knew what his life was like through viewing pictures on his phone, listening to him and his family, and reading to him, I actually knew very little about him." His funeral offered a much more expansive view of his humanity not defined by illness, chemotherapy, transfusions, and hospitalizations. I realized that the insight a healthcare team can gain about a patient through brief conversations in the hallway and through interdisciplinary meetings amount to just a few tiny pieces of an intricate puzzle depicting the rich and beautiful tapestry of a person's life. Despite our efforts, we still miss so much of the bigger picture. In the end, this invitation was the strong message that I needed to tell me that, despite my earlier misgivings, I had given this child and his family what they felt they needed. In the final analysis, I feel as though I did the right thing for him even though we never spoke about his fears of death, as his parents requested.

The End Lesson

One of the most enduring lessons I have learned by caring for gravely ill children is this: The parents we see are people who have come to us asking for help with their child. Wipe away everything else. The most we can do is offer them what we think will help them, their child, and the rest of their family. However, my job is not to convince them to accept my recommendations. My job is to meet them as a person and say, "This is how I think I can be helpful to you and your child." I tell them that honesty, transparency, and collaborative decision-making are the foundations of my practice. When parents receive information through this mode of communication, I trust them to make the best decision for themselves, their child, and their family—and that may mean they decide I cannot be helpful for them at this point in their child's illness. When that happens, I tell them that their decision sounds like the right one for them at this time, and if they ever change their minds they can always ask us to come back—because in the end, as much as my job is to empower children it is also to empower their parents.

For me, it's no longer about "saving" people. I think we sometimes stray off course when we have ideas about how we are going to save a child medically by offering chemotherapy, a stem cell transplant, or some other treatment. We clinicians have the tendency to think that it is our duty to save a child from a horrible death and save their family from the agony of seeing them die on a ventilator or on a dialysis machine by insisting on a "Do Not Resuscitate" order. Over the past few years, I have begun to realize the fallacy of those notions. Parents are not asking us to save them or their children. They are only asking us to help them. Maybe that help comes in the form of reading a book to their child for 30 minutes every day.

PRACTICE POINTS

Key Reflections

- Clinicians who have experienced significant illness can reflect on those experiences to better imagine their patients' feelings of helplessness, fear, grief, and sadness and thereby build their empathic abilities.

- Sick children who face the real prospect of death often develop a distorted picture of life, almost like half fantasy and half reality. As a result, hospitalized kids occupy a private world that adults cannot fully access or understand.

- When kids withhold access to their private world they exert what is arguably their last vestige of control, which is a normal and healthy way of preserving whatever identity and dignity they still possess.

- Parents view their primary role as protector, a role they feel they have not fulfilled if their child dies, even if that belief seems irrational to others.

- Parents of seriously ill children strike a sort of Faustian bargain: As their children become progressively more ill, they become increasingly willing to sacrifice their child's quality of life in hopes of achieving an ever more elusive cure.

- Parents of gravely ill children often ask clinicians not to speak frankly with their children about death.

- Many clinicians feel uncomfortable speaking honestly with gravely ill children about death, so they hide the truth, even though most children understand the gravity of the situation.

- Seriously ill children are often much more resilient than adults give them credit for.

- The view of a child's life that clinicians gain by caring for that child usually represents a mere sliver of that child's full humanity.

Empathic Actions

- When discussing a sensitive topic with a gravely ill child, a clinician should cede control of the conversation to the child to the extent possible.

- Giving a sick child total control over the patient-clinician relationship, at least in the beginning, often helps build trust in the relationship.

- Seriously ill children sometimes just need to feel like normal kids and forget about their circumstances for at least a few minutes every day. One way clinicians can help them achieve this goal is by speaking to them about their interests rather than about medical issues.

- Parents of sick children come to us asking for help with their children. We should wipe away everything else and realize that the most we can do is offer them what we think will help them, their children, and the rest of their family.

- Clinicians have the tendency to erroneously believe that it is their duty to save a child from a horrible death and to save their family from the agony of seeing them die on a ventilator or on a dialysis machine by insisting on a "Do Not Resuscitate" order. However, parents are not asking us to save them or their children but are instead only asking us for help.

- Many times a gesture as small as reading a book to a child for a few minutes rather than speaking about medical issues is the best way of demonstrating care and compassion.

Empathic Expression

- (Addressing a child who is rapidly approaching death): "Hey, I'm going to tell you some things that I *do not* think will scare you, because I have an idea you already know them."

- (Normalizing the situation): "I've worked with many kids who are in your situation, and they're often really scared if people haven't been honest with them or if they feel like people have kept information from them. Do you feel that way or have you ever felt that way?"

- "This is your opportunity to talk, but only if you want to. Do you want to tell me more? If you don't, that's okay. I don't need you to. But here's your opportunity to ask the questions that you probably are thinking about or want to know the answers to."

- "This is your home, and I am a guest in it. I don't want to spend any more time here than you find valuable. I don't want to waste your time."

- "Other kids who are in the hospital for a long time often wonder if they're getting sicker or whether they might die. Do you ever wonder that?"

- Sometimes a direct message is the most compassionate message: "If you want to be able to see him (the patient), you need to get him out of the hospital, and you have a very narrow window in which to do so."

- "If you want my help, this is how I can help you. I would love to work with you, but I completely understand if you want to take a different path. If you do, please remember to call us in the future if you think we may be able to help you."

10 | Only 4 of 6 Cycles

Oluchi C. Oke and Daniel E. Epner

HER WORDS LANDED like a hard slap across my face, but her tone was more resignation than anger: "I don't trust you." Queasiness welled up in my stomach. How can anyone not trust me? I am the consummate professional, attired in fashionable but not flashy clothing, understated jewelry and a starched white coat. My hair is always perfect. I sit at eye level, listen generously, and address my patients with respect and authenticity. I show up for work early and stay late, because my parents always said, "If you show up on time, you are late." I keep up with all the latest medical advances and treat all my patients with the utmost respect and compassion, whether rich or poor, Black or White. Perhaps most importantly, I am honest. I tell patients with stage IV cancer, "I am afraid your cancer is not curable", but then I quickly add, "But it is treatable." I epitomize trust, so I must have misheard my patient. I asked, "You don't trust me?" "That's right; I don't trust you or any of your people." I can understand why a few of my patients may wonder, "Does this young doctor have enough experience to take good care of me? Her name looks African. Did she train in America or in some foreign country?" However, their skepticism quickly melts away after they get to know me and find out that I trained at prestigious U.S. institutions. I take great pride in connecting with my patients, but I had obviously failed miserably with this woman. I needed to figure out a way to regain her trust.

She was a 50-year-old African-American woman with stage I breast cancer that was highly curable with standard therapy. However, she also had a lot of things happening in her life around the time of her cancer diagnosis. She had gotten married the week before and was supposed to have a honeymoon. Then all of a sudden, we told her, "You need six cycles of chemotherapy, surgery, radiation, and then Herceptin for a full year." Then on top of that, she lost her job due to the pandemic and was about to get a new job but had to attend to her health instead. She started a job for a couple of weeks but could not keep up her work schedule due to her many medical appointments. Despite her considerable psychosocial issues, I viewed her primarily through a medical lens: she was highly curable, and my main goal was to make her cancer a distant memory. Yes, I needed to connect with her on a human level, but she could always get another job later.

Passively Accepting Defeat

Most breast cancer patients are vigilant about treatment. Even the word "cancer" strikes fear in their hearts, so most patients will go to any length to achieve the best possible outcome, hopefully cure. Patients are so motivated that I often find myself trying to convince a woman that delaying chemotherapy for a week to allow her blood counts to recover is unlikely to reduce her chance of cure and is necessary to ensure her safety. Nearly all my patients are as aggressive as possible, but this woman was different from the start. She seemed reluctant and strangely passive, almost nonchalant, as if she was trying to avoid treatment. I saw her in my clinic the morning before her first cycle of chemotherapy and told her that her lab work looked fine and that she was ready to start treatment. Then she snuck out of the building without going to the infusion suite. When the nurse told me she had not shown up, I called her and asked, "Are you coming back for treatment?" She said, "I guess so." Her reply unnerved me. Did this woman understand that she was playing Russian roulette with her life? I thought, "How ironic that many cancer patients who are near death seek more treatment, hoping for a miracle, yet this woman was seemingly discarding her one good chance for cure." I rationalized, "She must fear possible side effects. I am sure she will come around after she finds out that chemotherapy is not so bad." Then, she tolerated treatment generally well, except for a bit more diarrhea than expected. Before cycle two, I explained how we would modify the doses slightly to reduce diarrhea, but her diarrhea paradoxically worsened instead. In addition, her neuropathy unexpectedly worsened even though we discontinued docetaxel. She did not understand or did not want to accept the premise that side effects like neuropathy can persist for a long time, even though we went to great lengths to explain this point. I also thought she may not want to wake up in time for an early infusion, but when I moved her appointment later the next cycle, she still came up with some excuse for being late. Despite all our education, accommodation, and encouragement, she missed her blood draw before cycle two, so we had to reschedule lab work repeatedly before she finally showed up. After two cycles of constant cajoling, I began to realize that her reluctance represented more than just normal misgivings about chemotherapy. The more we accommodated, the less she seemed to trust us, and the more she pushed us away. This lady was not fighting for her life like nearly every other patient. It was as if she was passively accepting defeat.

My Cancer Is Gone

My advanced practice provider (APP) and I somehow convinced her to complete four of the planned six cycles of induction chemotherapy by employing a kind of good cop, bad cop routine. Some weeks my APP called the patient with words of encouragement and support while I warned her about the grave consequences of not completing treatment, and then other weeks we switched roles. The woman's electronic health record is riddled with countless notes describing our phone encounters. Then her interim scan showed no residual disease, the best possible response, which steeled my determination to push forward with treatment. However, in my patient's mind the final two cycles of chemotherapy were unnecessary since the first four had apparently wiped out all her cancer. Her stance was confusing, because on the one hand she said, "I am cured, my cancer is gone" but on the other hand she sought alternative therapies in the community that her friend's dad was receiving for colon cancer. So, she clearly understood that she wasn't cured because she sought more treatments, but she kept saying, "The cancer is gone. Why do you need to give me more treatment and why do I need surgery?" She seemingly did not understand that there may still be subclinical tumor deposits in her body, either in her breast, at distant sites, or both. In addition, she complained that her side effects were worsening despite all the modifications we made to her chemotherapy.

A Question of Competence

Her approach to illness was so bizarre that I briefly wondered whether she suffered from mental illness. Nonetheless, I decided against involving psychiatry to assess her competence, because she seemed to know exactly what she was doing. She was very bright and had excellent health literacy and was never paranoid or delusional. Even when she said she thought the cancer was gone she clearly did not, because she sought alternative treatments. She also never perused the internet looking for information to refute our recommendations. She listened carefully to our explanations and recommendations and could repeat everything we said. I thought she may have adjustment disorder with anxiety as many cancer patients do, but she did not seem that anxious. I suppose she may have a personality disorder, but she never showed signs of one. She seemed to get along well with all the important people in her life. For instance, she often said her new husband was supportive and would give her rides to and from appointments and pick things up for her from the store. I also spoke to her husband by phone, and he described a healthy relationship with her. When I met her young adult daughter, they seemed to have a good relationship as well, joking with one another. She also got along well with children from her previous marriage and several friends. She was always very pleasant, never argumentative or antagonistic, but she would not budge no matter how we tried to convince her to finish treatment. I concluded that she was probably just overwhelmed by all the stressors in her life and that psychotropic medications and counseling would not reverse her persistent rejection of treatment.

Bartering Phase

After encouraging and accommodating her in every imaginable way, we went into full negotiation mode, almost as if we were bartering over a used car. When she politely insisted that we, "take this port out of my body," we offered to administer the final two cycles of chemotherapy through a peripheral IV. Then we said we would leave out the chemotherapy drug that caused diarrhea and just give her Herceptin, but she again failed to budge. After several unsuccessful attempts to get her back on the standard chemotherapy track, we reluctantly acquiesced and told her we could stop chemotherapy and send her directly for lumpectomy, hoping she would still have a good outcome even without the last two cycles. She said, "I don't want surgery, because everything you people said would happen to me either did not happen the way you said it would or was actually worse. Also, I don't want complications from surgery, even though you told me the complications are rare and usually not major." She had body image concerns, because she said, "I don't want to walk around without a breast if some unexpected complication happens during or after surgery." She would have undergone unilateral breast reconstruction, which was highly likely to proceed well, but she did not want to take the risk. I remember she said something about wanting her breasts to be even, so she requested a mastectomy rather than the customary lumpectomy. She calmly reiterated that she didn't trust us, which felt like the harshest blow. I would not have minded so much if she were a frail, elderly woman who weighed risks and benefits and decided to take a less aggressive stance, but she was curable.

A Matter of Race

After our attempts at accommodation, encouragement, and negotiation failed, I thought she may harbor a deep distrust of the American healthcare system, as many African-Americans do after experiencing centuries of societal inequity and injustice. I even mentioned this issue openly, but she just sat in silence and stared at her lap. Then I thought, "How can her distrust and resistance pertain to race? My nurse practitioner and I are both Black! Plus, I do not exactly epitomize the grave injustices of the Tuskegee experiment." I was born in Nigeria and moved to the United States when I was five when my dad got a Fulbright scholarship at UC Berkley and then joined the faculty as a professor of sociology at the University of Wyoming. We were the Ukaegbu family (pronounced OO-K-BOO) in Laramie, the land of Smiths, Johnsons, Millers, and Jones. We lived in the community for years before even a few of my classmates learned to pronounce my name correctly. Education was like the gold standard to my parents. My mom is still a nurse and nurse educator, and all five of my siblings are highly educated and professionally successful in a variety of fields. Even my given name distances me from systemic injustices in America. Oluchi means "God's work" in Igbo, a language spoken in Southern Nigeria. My mom was worried because back then in Nigeria no one was inducing labor and I was delivered almost 3 ½ weeks after my due date, so it was "God's work" that I finally arrived safely. In the final analysis, I concluded that my patient probably did not associate me with the American healthcare system as a whole and that her distrust of me had little to do with race.

"I'm Done"

During her clinic visit before her fifth cycle of chemotherapy, I resigned myself to the possibility that she would never finish treatment. I had tried encouragement, accommodation, bargaining, and even cajoling, all to no avail. I told her, "I can only imagine how you are feeling with the symptoms lingering and all the changes in your life. All this hit you so soon after you got married and started a new job. I will do whatever I can to improve your symptoms, but I desperately want you to be cured of your cancer." On the day of her fifth cycle, which we rescheduled for the weekend at her request, she checked in but did not answer when they called her to go back to the infusion suite. She was gone. I called her to ask where she was, and she said, "I'm done." I asked, "Did we keep you waiting too long? I apologize if we did. We can try to do better next time." She just repeated, "No, it's not that. I'm just done." She had hit the wall. She reached a breaking point, the perfect storm of side effects, fear of the future, life stressors, and body image concerns. Occasionally patients cut treatment short, but they still show up for checkups. Others transition their care to another institution for insurance reasons. She never even showed up for her plastic surgery appointment and she ignored their calls as she had ours. I have never seen anyone check out like she did.

I keep hoping she will materialize one day in clinic after she recharges emotionally, and I keep checking her electronic health record every few days, hoping a note will appear that documents her re-emergence. However, I only get radio silence. I have not seen or heard from her in over 3 months. I hope she does not wait a long time and then show up with advanced cancer, because by then it will be too late to cure her. Sometimes I lie awake at night second-guessing myself, wondering, "What could I have done differently to re-engage her and to earn her trust? Should I have adjusted her doses earlier in the treatment to address side effects? Should I have added another anti-diarrheal drug?" I do not think making those adjustments would have mattered.

I now realize that we build trusting relationships with our patients on a solid foundation of communication. The elements of each conversation are like drugs in a cancer treatment regimen that we need to constantly monitor and adapt to each patient's unique needs. Some patients need lower doses of certain drugs or modified regimens to compensate for advanced age or comorbidities in the same way that some patients need more time to express themselves than others do. All patients need accurate information about biomedical aspects of their illness and treatment, but some require more detail than others. All cancer patients experience negative emotions like fear, sadness, grief, and anger, but some require a higher dose of empathy than others do. Empathy is the glue that binds us to our patients. We can overdose patients on chemotherapy or opiates, but we can never overdose them on empathy. Empathy has an infinite therapeutic index.

Reflections in the Dark

"I do not trust you." Her words still haunt me sometimes as I lie awake at night, considering how I will respond if

I see her again. I may just sit in silence and wait for her to continue. Perhaps she will cry and say, "I am sorry. I almost never get emotional like this." Then I will say, "That's ok. I can understand why you feel utterly overwhelmed. Crying is completely normal under these circumstances. I can only imagine how rough this cancer ordeal has been for you, with everything going on in your life. You have demonstrated true grit through your treatments so far. I respect your independence and your desire to live how you see fit. I promise to take care of you as well as I possibly can and help you find another doctor if you prefer. I need nothing from you now other than to allow us to accompany you on this journey, wherever it leads. I want you to know that we will be here to support you anyway possible no matter what you decide and no matter what happens. We are on your side and will remain there forever." Then I drift off into peaceful sleep, knowing that I am trustworthy.

PRACTICE POINTS

Key Reflections

- Sometimes even the most compassionate, skilled, experienced, and well-meaning clinicians are unable to formulate a treatment plan that meets a patient's expectations. No one succeeds all the time.

- Under those rare circumstances, clinicians can be left with feelings of frustration, anxiety, and incompetence.

- Clinicians who are unable to meet a patient's expectations despite their best efforts and intentions should remember to focus on process rather than on outcomes by maintaining excellence in both biomedical and psychosocial domains of care.

Empathic Actions

- Dressing and behaving in a professional manner is one way that clinicians can show respect to patients and thereby build their trust.

- The most effective physicians are those who synergize with other members of the health care team, including nurses, advanced practice providers, administrative staff, and the psychosocial team.

- Spending extra time to thoroughly educate patients about risks and benefits of various treatment options and encouraging them to pursue the most beneficial path while avoiding coercion is one way that clinicians show they care.

Empathic Expression

- "I can only imagine how you are feeling with the symptoms lingering and all the changes in your life. All this hit you so soon after you got married and started a new job. I will do whatever I can to improve your symptoms, but I desperately want you to be cured of your cancer."

- "Did we keep you waiting too long? I apologize if we did. We can try to do better next time."

- "That's ok. I can understand why you feel utterly overwhelmed. Crying is completely normal under these circumstances."

- "I can only imagine how rough this cancer ordeal has been for you, with everything going on in your life."

- "You have demonstrated true grit through your treatments so far."

- "I respect your independence and your desire to live how you see fit."

- "I promise to take care of you as well as I possibly can and help you find another doctor if you prefer. I need nothing from you now other than to allow us to accompany you on this journey, wherever it leads."

- "I want you to know that we will be here to support you anyway possible no matter what you decide and no matter what happens. We are on your side and will remain there forever."

11 | Going the Extra Mile

Donna S. Zhukovsky and Daniel E. Epner

A PATIENT I cared for recently reminded me that actions can sometimes be more empathic than the most empathic words. The hospitalist asked me to see a man in the ICU with progressive refractory lung cancer who experienced respiratory failure and required mechanical ventilation. Prior to intubation, his dying wish was to return to his hometown, a 4–5-hour drive from our hospital. After compassionate extubation by the ICU team the day before, a Sunday, to prepare him for transition to hospice, his family was determined to get him back home no matter what. When I arrived on the scene a few minutes after receiving the consultation request, the man's family was so irate that they literally would not let me into the room to see him. Multiple daughters and granddaughters, some of whom were nurses with strong opinions about his care, filled the hallway, where they loudly directed a barrage of grievances toward me, barely pausing for breath. They were so angry and frustrated that I was unable to get meaningful information from them, so I stood there silently and allowed them to vent for several minutes. They eventually calmed down enough to explain that the ICU team had assured them that they could make the trip back home the next morning, only to find out that several logistical details were delaying discharge and making it increasingly likely that the man would die before making it home. To compound the problem, his family had already paid several thousand dollars for a ground ambulance that was non-refundable. The hospitalist coming on service that day asked our supportive care team to facilitate transition home to hospice at the 11th hour, even though we had never met the patient before.

After my initial hallway encounter with the family members, I excused myself to review his medical record in more detail and spoke with his hospitalist, case manager, ethicist, social worker, and the hospice medical director in his hometown who had accepted his care. After extubation the day before, the ICU team had implemented their typical comfort care orders, which included high-dose opioid and midazolam infusions. All with good intentions, the case manager, intensivist, and the previous hospitalist had arranged home hospice to meet the family's timeline, not understanding the intricacies and complexities this entailed. They were trying to discharge him home on midazolam and fentanyl infusions at doses that neither the hospitalist nor I were comfortable prescribing. In addition, no one had adequately addressed several practical details, such as how the ambulance crew would administer infusions in transit or where the pumps would be obtained for the infusions, since our pharmacy was unable to send hospital pumps with him. Other reasons for concern included the high doses of both medications and the hospice agency's ability and willingness to continue them in the home hospice setting. After my initial evaluation, I told the family that we would do everything in our power to get him home as quickly as possible that day, but wanted to do so in a way that would ensure a smooth transition without risk of return to the hospital and that I would update them shortly with a plan. They reluctantly acknowledged the issues I discussed with them and displayed somewhat less distress.

I then moved a short distance away so as to minimize distractions and formulate a plan while his family remained clustered in the hallway outside his room. I was relieved to learn from the patient's wife that he had not experienced much pain before hospital admission or during hospitalization, so I was uncertain why an opioid infusion was started in the first place. On the bright side, I concluded that he would likely need little, if any, pain medicine during his journey home in the ambulance and would certainly not require a constant infusion. Luckily, the hospitalist had placed a fentanyl patch on that morning so we had a head start on his analgesic regimen. I also found out that his initial delirium was attributable to hypercalcemia; at present, he only got agitated when he wanted to stand up to urinate. Accordingly, I was not particularly worried about high levels of agitation and thought he would require minimal if any sedation on the way home. We decided to discontinue the midazolam infusion and replace it with lorazepam only as needed, which the ambulance personnel could administer by syringe during the trip home. Appropriate dosing required knowledge of conversion ratios of the different benzodiazepines, which was not readily available, so I contacted our pharmacist and a psychiatry colleague for advice. In the final analysis, I concluded that he did not need an infusion of pain medicine or sedative during the ambulance ride home, so we sent him home with a modest number of lorazepam and fentanyl syringes for use in transit if needed, after expediting their preparation with the hospital pharmacy. The next step was to involve case management to ensure that there were ambulance staff who were qualified to administer IV medication during the trip home. Last, but not least, I called the hospice medical director in his home city to discuss the change in plan and establish her readiness to accept his care. This process of weighing options and coordinating with colleagues took well over an hour, but I now had a workable plan to present to the family.

I then returned to the patient's room, at which point the gauntlet of concerned family members standing sentry in the hallway parted to allow me to enter, where the man's wife and son-in-law awaited me. I explained that we had done our best to anticipate as many glitches as possible to ensure his trip home went as seamlessly as possible. I then asked the man's wife and son-in-law to call the rest of the family back in the room. After giving each an opportunity to express their grievances, questions and concerns, I then summarized the plan and the process by which I had developed it. I also acknowledged their distress and apologized for any misinformation they had received, explaining that I was consulted shortly before meeting them and after they had made their plan. They moved on to express their gratitude for helping them fulfill their loved one's wishes and supporting them in their goal to get him home that day. The patient left by ambulance a short time later accompanied by his wife and trailed by his family members in their own cars. A call the next day let us know that he had made it home safely and was lovingly surrounded by his extended family and friends.

As I look back on this scenario, it is easy to see that my actions spoke much more loudly than any empathetic words could have. In fact, I spent much of my time with the family just listening to their grievances before springing into action to develop a plan that required complex relational skills, biomedical knowledge, and experience to meet the family's acute needs. Taking a detailed history and dotting the i's and crossing the t's to conform to our typical comprehensive palliative care consultation for this man would have been wrong for this family. They desperately wanted to respect his dying wish and needed me to take decisive action if they were to succeed. I could have said many classically empathic statements including the words "I wish…" and "I cannot imagine…," but they probably would have fallen on deaf ears in light of the family's anger and frustration. Ultimately, what made them happy was getting him home to his own bed.

PRACTICE POINTS

Key Reflections

- Decisive action on behalf of the patient and family can be more empathic than even the most empathic words.

- Clinicians need to imagine what the patient and family are experiencing in order to take empathic action.

- Anger is an external manifestation of underlying negative emotions, such as fear, anxiety, grief, or sadness.

- Silent presence to allow people to vent their anger and frustration for a few minutes is often very therapeutic.

- Forging healing relationships with patients and their families requires not just excellent communication and interpersonal skills, but also outstanding technical skills and knowledge.

Empathic Actions

- One way that clinicians show patients they care is by coordinating closely with other teams through phone calls and electronic communication to make sure everyone is on the same page.

- Even the most knowledgeable clinicians often need to take the time to seek biomedical information from evidence-based sources or colleagues to ensure that they are making sound medical decisions.

- Empathic clinicians sometimes need to take actions that are beyond their job descriptions to accomplish important goals for their patients.

Empathic Expression

- Family: The case manager told us the hospitalist would discharge him this morning, but we just found out the ambulance is not ready to take him. We already spent $10,000 on the ambulance, and now it looks like we are going to lose our money!

  - Traditional response:

    - I am going to defer to the case manager regarding logistical questions.

  - **Recommended empathic responses:**

    - I can see how important it is for you to get your husband home.

    - I do not blame you for feeling frustrated with this process. I would feel frustrated too if I were in your shoes. I still think we can get your husband ready for discharge in time to ride the ambulance you paid for.

- Family: I am sorry I blew up at you before. I was worried I would lose the money I paid for the ambulance and would not be able to get my husband home as I promised.

  - Traditional response:

    - Apology accepted

  - **Recommended empathic responses:**

    - You do not need to apologize. I know your words came from a place of love and that you were only trying to advocate for your husband.

    - I respect how strongly you are advocating for your husband and the rest of your family.

    - To patient's daughter: I can see how much you love your father. He must be a great father.

12 Just Do What You Do

Reverend Asa W. Roberts Jr. and
Daniel E. Epner

As a chaplain in the Palliative Care Department at MD Anderson Cancer Center, I work closely with doctors, nurses, and other clinicians every day. As a result, I constantly witness the many ways in which clinicians forge strong, healing relationships with vulnerable patients, and I see many parallels between the work that they do and my work as a spiritual adviser. Seriously ill patients see clinicians as much more than technical experts who diagnose and treat disease. They also expect their doctors and other clinicians to transcend traditional clinical roles and practice with great humanism. My role as a chaplain is well defined: I work purely in the spiritual domain. However, the lines blur for clinicians, who straddle the biomedical, psychosocial, and spiritual domains. I therefore believe that my work as a chaplain is highly relevant to the everyday practice of empathic clinicians.

Spirituality in My DNA

I come from a family of ministers and pastors, including my father, grandfather, and several uncles and cousins. My father first entered the ministry in Detroit when he was still working full time for the postal service. After working both jobs for a while, he decided to pursue ministry full time, so he moved our family from our comfortable and stable life in Detroit to a little town outside of Pittsburgh called Aliquippa. His position at the church in Aliquippa paid very little, so we went from living in our own nice house in Detroit to living in public housing, which was an experience that was hard for my three sisters and me to navigate, truly beyond words. I was just a third-grader at the time, and I was thinking, "I can't believe we're doing this." My father had taken a huge leap of faith in order to pursue his calling. Fortunately, as he continued to nurture his commitment to religion, he got an offer to lead a larger church in another suburb of Pittsburgh four years later, which allowed me to witness the power of faith. His income was much greater than it had been in the previous position, so we soon got our own house again. Thank God for resolving our housing situation.

Besides working full time as a Pastor in his church, my father also brought formal religion into our home by continuing a family tradition that my grandfather started. He gathered our entire family around the table for Sunday morning devotion each week before we went to church. The rule of the house was that no matter how late we stayed out on Saturday night, we would have to get up and be at the table by 7 am for full devotion. My dad always cooked a big breakfast and read Scripture, and everyone in the family had to pray. My father had seven siblings, and I can remember times when several cousins were in town on holiday and 20 or more people would attend Sunday devotion, with kids lined up our staircase. I might have been bleary-eyed through several of these Sunday morning family devotions after a late night, but they were nonetheless an important part of my foundation in spirituality and religion. Spirituality is in my DNA.

My father ultimately attained high moral stature in the community and served on the boards of several prominent institutions, including Penn State University. He served as pastor of his church for 53 years before retiring in 2014 at the age of 95. When he died in 2017, the city named the street in front of his church after him. He was a tremendous role model. In retrospect, my father clearly wanted me to follow his example and enter the ministry. However, he never pressured me to do so, even though I am his only son and his namesake. He often told me to, "Just do what you do," in other words, "Follow your own path." As a result, I decided not to enter the ministry despite the fact that it was an honorable profession, because I had witnessed all the hardships my father and other relatives endured with their congregations.

A Career in Business and a Calling in the Ministry

After my father gave me his blessing to pursue a path other than the ministry, I studied business in college, got an MBA, and entered the oil and gas business. As I moved up the corporate ranks, I moved throughout the United States and also lived in several foreign countries. After many years of success in the oil and gas business, I remember calling my dad one day to tell him that my family and I were doing well personally and professionally, but that something was still missing in my life and that I could not fill the void despite my outward success.

Around that time, my mother died, and my father asked that I speak for the family at her funeral. I told him, "I am happy to do so, but keep in mind that I am a speaker, not a preacher." He replied with his common refrain, "Just do what you do." A short time later, we spoke again by phone and he told me he would have an anniversary as minister of his church within a few months and asked if I would be willing to address his congregation to honor the occasion. I said, "Whoa that is really out of my league. I told you I am a speaker not a preacher," at which point he again said, "That is fine. Just do what you do." Therefore, I spoke in front of his congregation on the anniversary of his Ministry. Even though I repeatedly said I was not a preacher, the more I spoke at his church on special occasions, the more I wrapped my words with scripture. About three months later, I had an epiphany, and when I returned home, I asked my father if I could take a few minutes to make an announcement in front of the congregation. He agreed, and I told everyone that, effective that moment, I was a preacher not a speaker. I had accepted the calling that lay buried deep within me my whole life. My father must have smiled knowingly hearing my words. One of his favorite sayings was, "God can run you down standing still." I never understood what those words meant the many times I heard them when I was growing up. However, after experiencing my own spiritual awakening, I finally understood that he meant that God is so powerful he can guide a person to a righteous life even if he tries to run in the other direction. Standing on the altar that day, my mindset changed dramatically. I applied myself to religion and spirituality as eagerly as I had applied myself to the business world. I shifted gears suddenly and attended divinity school, then got a Master's degree followed by a doctorate. A preacher was born, but only after a long, winding journey.

Young Patients Hit Me the Hardest

I have always been able to deal with what I call the D trilogy: death, dying, and despair, because I witnessed death at a young age. For instance, some teenagers who went to my high school died in a car accident when I was a sophomore or junior, and one of my good friends in school died when he was about 14. However, those deaths were outside my family, so they did not hit me that hard. My youngest sister's death, on the other hand, touched me deeply, and I still think of her often when I minister to young patients. She died of some type of liver disease at age 20 or 21. At the time, liver transplants were rare, so she did not get one. She was a clean-living girl who acquired a random, unexplainable disease and died for no good reason. She was truly an innocent victim. After she died, my parents told us that the doctors did not expect her to live long enough to graduate from high school, although my two other sisters and I were kept in the dark all those years. We knew she was tired all the time during her teen years, but we did not make much of it. In fact, I remember being annoyed on occasion when my parents treated her with kid gloves, since I concluded she must have been getting preferential treatment as the youngest child. Later, after her death, my two other sisters and I wondered why our parents had not told us about her condition when she was still alive. Even though my father served as a wise spiritual leader for our community, he was a grieving parent like any other and therefore probably had no idea what to tell us about my sister's illness and impending death. In retrospect, I can only imagine the misery my parents must have experienced as my sister dwindled. Nonetheless, I wish they had allowed my other sisters and me to share in their fear and grief so we could have nurtured my sister and fully cherished the limited time we had with her. If they had, I would have sat by her side, held her hand, hugged her, told her how much I loved her, and exchanged stories. I would have asked her how she wanted people to remember her and I would have encouraged her to create art and write letters, poems, and stories that would live after her body gave out. My sister's memory burns inside me and informs my practice every day, especially when I see young patients.

A Young Man with a Chaotic Childhood

I thought of my sister recently when I ministered to a young man in his early 20s, although his background was nothing like ours. He grew up in a very dysfunctional family and his parents divorced when he was a young child, after which he was raised by his mother and stepfather for a while, and then raised by an uncle. He bounced around from one unstable, chaotic environment to another and spent a considerable part of his childhood essentially living on the streets in horrible neighborhoods amongst drug dealers and other unsavory characters. He struggled mightily in school and displayed the expected behavioral problems, yet many of his teachers nonetheless noticed that he was academically gifted in many subjects. He somehow managed to compose poetry and create art amongst all the chaos with support from teachers, one of whom welcomed him into his family. He got an academic scholarship to college where he shared an apartment with three other young men whose families were instrumental in supporting him and providing a positive influence. For instance, he sometimes stayed with them to celebrate major holidays. Then, just as he was turning his life around, he developed an aggressive form of cancer.

One of the biggest challenges I face is when patients will not open up to me. During the months before I met this young man, he met two other chaplains and was engaging during both of those encounters. In fact, at the end of the first of those visits, he expressed fear and did not want the chaplain to leave. About a month later, he had a similarly productive meeting with the second chaplain. However, those meetings occurred while he was still receiving treatment for his cancer and maintained hope for a positive outcome. By the time I met him, this young man had already experienced a series of peaks and valleys, successes and failures and had just received news from the treating team that they could no longer treat his cancer. As a result, he was subdued and clammed up when I entered his room. He refused to engage but instead internalized everything, often responding with one word answers or complete silence.

The Power of Presence

After I had difficulty connecting with him during our initial meetings, I collaborated with one of the other chaplains during my visit to see if I could connect with him. However, he still rejected our outreach and asked that we return another time. Later when we returned, he mumbled a few words unintelligibly and turned away from us. I kept returning periodically, and sometimes I would enter his room to find him lying there as though he were sleeping. For the first few such encounters, I left his room after several seconds if he did not awaken. However, I eventually decided to be more persistent, so I sat down even when he appeared to be asleep and carried on a one-sided conversation. When I did, he finally opened his eyes and said, "I am a little sleepy now," which gave me an opening to talk about his sleepiness and discuss how some medications can cause sleepiness, all the while knowing that his silence was attributable to depression more than it was related to sedation. If nothing else, I was persistent in maintaining a physical presence at his side.

I also tried to engage him by restating questions in different ways or reflecting by saying something like, "I noticed you didn't respond when I asked that question about your background and your upbringing." I carefully observed his body language and sometimes said, 'I noticed you appeared anxious when I asked about your background. Are you upset about something you or someone else did or something else about your past?" I also asked, "Do you want to discuss some unresolved issues?" I asked a series of questions to encourage him to tell his story.

The Silent Companion

I call this practice of encouraging patients to open up and tell their stories the silent companion approach, which involves posing open-ended questions, sitting silently to receive whatever information the patient wants to share, and letting the patient take the conversation wherever he or she wants. My spiritual teachers always trained me to meet people wherever they are, which means discussing a person's faith, regardless of what that faith is, or supporting people who have a spiritual connection to something other than religion. For instance, some people connect with pets, like their dogs, because their dogs love them unconditionally, regardless of whether the day is sunny, rainy, or chilly. I learn where someone is and then affirm that place, which allows me to help people of any faith or even people for whom spiritual or religious faith is not a primary source of peacefulness. Taking this stance allows me to meet them wherever they are, affirm them, and try to connect and travel with them on their journey. In other words, I encourage people to "do what they do," as my father would say.

The clinicians I admire the most are those who integrate the silent companion approach into their conversations with patients. Some people may consider therapeutic listening to be passive, but in reality listening effectively is very active and requires nuanced skills. Besides taking the obvious steps of avoiding distractions and using attentive body language, the clinicians who I believe are most effective also briefly summarize what the patient says during momentary breaks in the conversation in a way that demonstrates comprehension of the *essence* of the story while not interrupting the flow of ideas. This process requires insight into subtle and often hidden meanings of words that are communicated through tone and cadence as well as close attention to nonverbal cues communicated by facial expression and body language. So, the power of presence applies equally well to clinicians and chaplains. In the final analysis, all people have a need to be heard, especially those who are scared and vulnerable.

The Chaplain's Job: Bring Spirituality into the Conversation

Despite my efforts to engage the young man, he steadfastly refused to open up, even though he was still clear-headed and could have conversed if he wanted to. I therefore decided to build upon the silent companion model by introducing various metaphors that relate to religion and spirituality. I first tried the wounded healer metaphor that involves describing experiences in my life that pertain to the patient's situation. For instance, I explained to him that I have been under-appreciated or rejected at times in my life, and I then waited to see if my message resonated. My goal was to lift him up and move him to a better emotional state, but he still did not budge. I then played the role of a gardener who suggests, "Clipping some of the branches from your tree" to help him gain perspective and get rid of excess baggage, such as people in his orbit who might do or say things that are harmful to him. This too did not resonate with him.

As expected, the young man had no access to organized religion as a child because of his chaotic upbringing, but had committed himself to Christ in recent years and underwent baptism as a nondenominational Christian. However, when I saw him as he approached the end of his life, he had reversed course, felt as though God had abandoned him, and understandably began to doubt his faith commitment. I could only imagine his life, raising himself in a dangerous and chaotic environment, eventually attracting support and stewardship from his church and school, and feeling as though he had finally gotten on the right track and had broken the cursed generational cycle. Then, the cancer came down hard on his head and hovered over him like a dark cloud. I told him, "I can't explain why any of this happened: your rough childhood, your cancer, or your failing health. I cannot understand it and I do not have an answer. I cannot imagine how you must feel or how difficult your journey has been." Then I turned to spirituality.

"Please remember, the God who guided you to success is the same God who is still in control and still loves you. No one really knows what happens to us after we leave this earth, but if you believe in Heaven as I do, then you should begin to think about where you go from here." As a spiritual leader, I want people to think beyond their physical beings. I tried to connect on several different levels. I continued to try to get some family members to visit, because he was longing for a relationship with his mother. Unfortunately, she was preoccupied using drugs and pursuing all the dysfunctional activities she had pursued his whole life, so she abandoned him at his time of greatest need.

Some people may think that introducing spirituality into a conversation with a patient is either presumptuous or coercive, since such conversations can be very difficult for patients who face existential crises. However, chaplains who discuss spirituality and religion without explicit permission from the patient are no more coercive or presumptuous than clinicians who feel the need to discuss goals of care or code status with seriously ill patients. Such sensitive conversations are necessary at times. Clinicians and spiritual leaders should certainly meet people where they are, as my father frequently encouraged me to do, but we often need to take the initiative to do more. Sometimes the most challenging conversations are the most important ones.

Despite the fact that I introduced spirituality into our conversations, the young man remained disengaged. However, he had not asked me to leave his room or asked to see another chaplain, so I concluded I must have made some progress. I then asked him if he was angry with God, which finally got his attention, because he turned toward me, sat up a little, and looked directly into my eyes. After thinking for several seconds, he shook his head "no." My first impulse was to tell him that I did not believe him, but I instead said, "I am surprised, because if I were in your shoes, I would be angry at God and I would be angry at many other people too." He remained silent, so after a few seconds I continued, "It is ok if you are angry with God. You can tell me you are, because God can handle it. God has broad shoulders and can carry the load." He remained quiet, but I had nonetheless engaged him to some extent, so I began to discuss the Psalms, specifically the life of David. I often point people to the Psalms, because they are songs of prayer, praise, and love that take people to a new point of orientation, a new perspective on life. The Psalms have movements that are symbolic of our own lives as we move from one orientation to another, such as when we move from a happy place where everything is ok to a place where everything seems to spiral down. I thought if this young man was angry with God and others around him, as he appeared to be, the Psalms could help him suddenly emerge from the depths, get a fresh start, realize his life has not been in vain, and move forward, even if for a short time before death. I tried to encourage him, because part of my role is to provide hope. I wanted to give him reasons to have hope, either in this life or the one after. Ideally, patients can verbalize their hopes and dreams, but when they cannot, I sometimes proactively inject hope into the conversation, in keeping with my role as a preacher. When I speak of the Psalms, I usually refer to Psalm 23, 91, or 27. As I recall, I recited excerpts from Psalm 91:

> *Thou shalt not be afraid of the terror by night; nor of the arrow that flies by day; nor of the pestilence that walks in darkness; nor of the destruction that wastes at noonday. A thousand shall fall at thy side and ten thousand at thy right hand; but it shall not come near thee....Thou has made the most High thy habitation. No evil shall befall thee, nor shall any plague come near thy dwelling. For he shall give his angels charge over thee, to keep thee in all thy ways.*

Psalm 91 talks about how God hides vulnerable people under his wings, just as a mama duck protects her ducklings from predators as they sit at the edge of the pond. I believe there is always some reason to live and to learn that the way in which we live our lives, our legacy, is our most important attribute. I wanted this young man to know that he should maintain his faith even under the direst circumstances and look beyond his failing body to where he may be going. I could never really tell what he thought of my words, since he remained subdued throughout our relationship. Nonetheless, I knew that I had tried everything in my power to bring healing to this young man's soul in his time of greatest need in ways that so few others ever had. I served as his silent companion, his wounded healer, his gardener who suggested "clipping some branches from his tree," and finally his bearer of Psalms. I only pray I succeeded in some small measure.

Ultimately, his condition deteriorated to the point where he could barely speak even if he had wanted to. His body had finally given out. The last time I saw him, I sat in silence by his bed for a while and then returned to Psalm 91, *"Thou shalt not be afraid of the terror by night... A thousand shall fall at thy side and ten thousand at thy right hand; but it shall not come near thee...."* As I did, I envisioned a mother duck protecting her ducklings with her outstretched wing. I then strained as hard as I could to envision God nurturing this young man's soul in Heaven, but the vision eluded me. After I finished reciting the entire Psalm, I paused and listened for a response, but he lay still and silent. When I offered to read another of his favorite passages, he finally summoned the few wisps of strength remaining in his body to open his eyes slightly, turn his head toward me, and say through labored breaths, "Thank you Reverend." He then mumbled words that I could not quite decipher, but they sounded like, "I want to rest now and spend time with...." His words trailed off into silence as he fell back to sleep. As I gazed upon him, I saw my baby sister once again, but now smiling broadly, appearing many years older than she did in life but entirely healthy, smiling radiantly. I then reached over to gently caress the young man's forehead and told him "Just do what you do."

PRACTICE POINTS

Key Reflections

- Seriously ill patients see clinicians as much more than technical experts who diagnose and treat disease. They also expect their doctors and other clinicians to transcend traditional clinical roles and practice with great humanism.

- Many clinicians consider medicine to be a higher calling to which they devote their lives in the service of their patients and society, just as religious leaders see their work as a calling in the service of God, their congregants, and humanity.

- A spiritual leader's service to God and an empathic clinician's service to patients both require devotion, discipline, and sacrifice.

- Spiritual advisers and clinicians have much to learn from one another.

- Memorable events in the lives of spiritual leaders and empathic clinicians, whether those events are joyful or sorrowful, profoundly impact the ways in which spiritual leaders and empathic clinicians carry out their work.

- In the final analysis, dignity and legacy are arguably a person's most valuable possessions.

Empathic Actions

- One of the basic tenets of spiritual practice is meeting people where they are by letting them "do what they do," much as one of the basic tenets of empathic medical practice is adapting to the unique needs of each patient.

- All people have a fundamental need to be heard.

- Generous listening is far from a passive process, but rather involves integrating silence in the right measure, avoiding interruptions, using attentive body language, and briefly interjecting a few words or phrases that demonstrate understanding of the essence of what the speaker is saying.

- Chaplains are often obligated to introduce religion and spirituality into conversations in an attempt to help patients find emotional and spiritual peace, just as clinicians are often obligated to broach sensitive topics, like goals of care and code status, even when patients are hesitant to discuss them.

Empathic Expression

- "Just do what you do."

- Exploratory statements to elicit narrative:

  ○ "I noticed you appeared anxious when I asked about your background. Are you upset about something you or someone else did or something else about your past?"

  ○ "Do you want to discuss some unresolved issues?"

- "Of course you are sleepy. Some of the medications you are taking cause sleepiness, which is not your fault."

- "Sometimes, people have to 'clip some of the branches from their tree' to get rid of excess baggage, such as people in their orbit who might do or say things that are harmful to them."

- "Please remember, the God who guided you to success is the same God who is still in control and still loves you.

No one really knows what happens to us after we leave this earth, but if you believe in Heaven as I do, then you should begin to think about where you go from here."

- "If I were in your shoes, I would be angry at God and I would be angry at many other people too. It is ok to be angry with God. You can tell me you are, because God can handle it. God has broad shoulders and can carry the load."

13 | Art Imitates Life*

Kimberson C. Tanco and Daniel E. Epner

I WAS ON the ESPN website the other day when I saw a video of JJ Watt announcing his plans to seek employment with a new team after playing with the Houston Texans for 10 years. For the few people who have not heard of JJ Watt, he is a perennial NFL all-pro and 3-time NFL defensive player of the year. "I sat down with [the ownership group], and we have mutually agreed to part ways." He then started to say how well everyone has treated him in Houston: "The way you guys have treated me…." He then paused for a moment to carefully consider his next words: "…besides draft night. You booed me on draft night, but every day after that you treated me like family." As I watched JJ deliver an inconvenient truth about the cruel reception he received on draft night, it occurred to me that we clinicians can learn a lot from his words. The truth is not always pretty, but we are obligated to tell it. JJ then continued by saying how grateful he was to be loved and supported by the organization, fans, teammates, friends, and community, and concluded with,

---

Kimberson Tanco is a Palliative Care doctor at MD Anderson Cancer Center.

"Thank you Houston, I love you." With just a few words, JJ showed how truth sometimes should be tempered with love and compassion. Oscar Wilde said, "Life imitates Art." However, for empathic clinicians, the art of medicine sometimes imitates the lives of world-class athletes.

99 Jersey Framed on the Wall

During a recent virtual video visit with a patient with metastatic cancer, I noticed a framed JJ Watt jersey hanging on the wall behind him. I had never met the patient, so I introduced myself as usual and said, "Wow, I noticed you have a framed JJ Watt jersey hanging on the wall behind you along with several other mementos. You have a very nice collection there." He said, "Oh, yeah, thanks." Then we started talking about Watt's potential future as a free agent.

I started: "Man, I sure am going to miss seeing him play for the Texans. He is the face of the organization. He has had a Hall of Fame career, but he hasn't gotten a championship ring yet. While I hate to see him go, I suppose he's making the right decision to join a team he thinks can win the Super Bowl. Where do you think JJ will end up next season?"

He replied: "I think he will try to join his brothers in Pittsburgh."

"Yes, I suppose so, but I think he would prefer to play for Green Bay so he can return to Wisconsin, where he grew up and played college ball."

He said, "I can't argue with that. Especially since he would get to play with one of the greatest quarterbacks of all time in Green Bay. Of course, in Houston he played with a great rising star in Deshaun Watson, but it looks like Deshaun may move soon too. So, it will be interesting to see what JJ decides."

We then carried on like this for a couple of minutes, discussing various personnel changes on the Texans in recent years and prospects for the future. I never overtly disagreed with him about any of his views, but we did not exactly agree about everything either. We had what one could characterize as an authentic but respectful exchange between two acquaintances in a sports bar or between friends sitting in front of the TV at home. The last thing I wanted was for him to think I was patronizing him. Then after reaching a natural lull in the conversation about football, we talked about his symptoms and other medical issues in a free-flowing fashion. The visit went very smoothly. We partnered in adjusting his analgesic regimen, and he seemed to trust me implicitly. He was very appreciative despite his considerable symptom burden and poor prognosis. A casual observer may have considered our opening conversation about football a frivolous waste of time. However, in reality, I think our conversation about everyday life helped create a meaningful connection between us very quickly the first time we met. When clinicians speak to patients like they would a friend or family member, even briefly, they reduce the power imbalance that invariably exists between them, recognize their patients' humanity rather than just their diagnoses and symptoms, and show they care.

Humor as a Form of Empathy

I have a patient who is Filipino like I am who I have gotten to know well over the past several months while caring for him in our outpatient clinic. I feel as though we have a very close relationship, almost like family. One day a few months ago, he presented to clinic sporting a half-grown mustache, so I half-jokingly told him how impressed I was by his new facial hair and how macho he looked. He said, "Well, you know, I want to be macho masunurin." In the Philippines, we have this word "masunurin," which means "obedient" as humorously applied to being obedient to your wife. So he did a little play on words with macho and masunurin, which was even funnier since his wife accompanied him to the visit, as she always does. Now we have a running joke between us so that every time I see him, I ask

"So how is Mr. Macho doing today?" Of course, after joking for a few minutes, we always attend fully to his medical needs.

I am not an expert on what makes something funny and how to best use humor to bond with patients. However, in this case, I think humor worked for a few reasons. First, the patient initiated playful, slightly self-deprecating humor to make light of his grave situation. He is dealing with all the effects of advanced cancer and he knows what the endpoint will be, but he and his wife need occasional moments of reprieve from the weight of his illness. Second, I think when I first mentioned his new mustache, I focused on something personal rather than medical and gave him a lighthearted compliment by calling him "macho" without trivializing his considerable medical issues. His humor was also therapeutic because it touched on our common cultural and linguistic backgrounds. I suppose anyone can see the humor of "macho masunurin," but I got the joke immediately and saw parallels in my life and in my parent's long marriage, in which my mother is also a source of strength. In the final analysis, I think listening carefully, following a patient's cues, and imagining a patient's and family's experiences—the essence of empathic practice—are the keys to using humor in a healing way.

Modeling Resilience

In my family, we tend to adapt to whatever comes our way and take everything in stride. My dad developed cancer when he was only 39, and he remains a cancer survivor over 30 years later. He needed several surgeries to treat recurrent cancer for the first 15 years, until about age 54. With each recurrence, he always said, "Well, this might be it for me. This may be my time." And he always seemed at peace with dying of cancer, saying, "I am ok with whatever happens." So he would carry on a normal life between bouts of cancer. He was a builder, so he would stop working during cancer treatment but would get right back at it after he recovered. He never just sat down and waited to die or let the cancer dominate his existence.

His illness never restricted us. We took trips, ate out, and basically lived a normal family life whenever he was well enough to do so. He remains a cancer survivor in remission even now, at age 72. I think watching my dad take everything in stride by not letting cancer become a dark cloud hanging over his head molded me and my approach to my patients. I often find myself expressing respect for patients who are resilient like my dad and live each day to its fullest. I also appreciate how resilient caregivers can be, since I saw my mom do everything to care for my dad when he was down, like monitoring his medications and side effects while taking care of our household and working first as a school teacher and later as a stockbroker. She handled all that stress with composure and good humor. "Mr. Macho" and his wife remind me of my parents and others I know, even though my parents are a few years older.

Respecting the Caregiver

When I see Mr. Macho in clinic, I often speak with his wife as much as I speak with him. I can sense that being the primary caregiver for a man to whom she has been married for four decades is extraordinarily stressful. She carries the weight of worrying about his condition and what they both know will be an unfavorable outcome. So, she jokes around at times, but she tends to remain serious most of the time so she can be effective as his caregiver. She always seems to be in thinking mode to ensure that she understands all my recommendations and that she can carry them out fully. I think a little humor lightens the atmosphere and helps her feel comfortable posing whatever questions she has.

I also think respecting her role as caregiver, wife, and mother is empathic and strengthens the bond between us. During Mr. Macho's most recent visit to our clinic, we modified his analgesic regimen and started a new medication for insomnia. Mr. Macho's wife then asked several questions to confirm the changes, and said, "Dr. Tanco, I am sorry to ask so many questions, but I want to make sure I get this right."

"Please, no need to apologize," I said. "I can see how much you love him."

She looked at me in silence for a few seconds and started to cry. "Our 40th anniversary is coming up in a few months. Our kids plan to visit to help us celebrate."

I thought about my mother's efforts caring for my father and spoke from my heart: "You are doing an amazing job caring for him. I respect how you always advocate for your husband. I also think that both of you have done a great job raising your children, based on what I know about them. Raising nice children is no small feat."

Mr. Macho started to tear up too. "Well, I think we got lucky with our kids. They're both good people who have given us beautiful grandchildren."

"You may be lucky to have such wonderful children, but I think you have also set a great example and have raised them right. Your role as parents and grandparents is arguably the most important part of your legacy. From what I can tell from prior conversations, you also treat your employees like family, so you can feel confident that your legacy is secure, regardless of how long you live."

Mr. Macho and his wife processed my words silently for a few seconds, thanked me, and left the room arm in arm. I think my words of respect and validation were more healing than any analgesic or sleeping pill I could have prescribed.

Joking and talking about everyday things with Mr. Macho and his wife feels natural, since we share a common nationality and language. Talking to the patient with the framed JJ Watt jersey about NFL free agents or with other patients about their favorite sports teams also seems natural, since I am a passionate sports fan. However, most of my patients are not Filipino, and many have no interest in sports. I therefore try to connect with everybody about topics that interest them, even if I know nothing about those topics. For instance, I know nothing about quilting other than that a big quilting expo takes place in Houston every year, or at least it did before the pandemic.

A 70-year-old woman who I saw in clinic not long ago even displayed her handiwork there in the past. When she told me about her hobby, my first instinct was to validate her by saying something like, "Oh that sounds fascinating! What a wonderful hobby!" However, I wanted to encourage more expression rather than end the conversation, so I asked, "What do you like most about quilting?" This was a woman who was severely diminished by cancer and its treatment, appearing frail and subdued. However, when I asked about quilting she tapped into a hidden reserve of energy and passion deep in her soul:

> *I remember the very first time I worked on a quilt. I was five years old, staying with my older brother at my grandma and grandpa's farm in Navasota County for the summer. Grandma, Aunt Martha, two cousins, my brother, and I crowded around the kitchen table designing our quilt for that year's county fair. My brother and I were too young to handle scissors or a needle and thread, so our job was to fetch swatches of cloth from the closet and deliver them to the kitchen for the ladies to consider, and then run them back to the closet when they were done. They probably could have brought all the samples out and stacked them on the kitchen counter ahead of time, but I suppose they wanted us to feel useful. We drank homemade lemonade and joked and gossiped late into the night, way past my bedtime. As I got older, I got more and more involved with cutting and sewing and finally got to design my own patterns. Later, I crowded around my own kitchen table with my mother, children, and other relatives designing quilts for the big Houston Expo and county fairs. In recent years I have had my grandkids out to our ranch for a few weeks each summer, and we work on quilts together just like we did when I was a little girl. Letting my grandkids work on quilts, tend to the animals, and do other chores around the ranch is the only way we can get them to put down their computers and phones for a little while.*

Feeding off Each Other

JJ Watt announced plans to join the Arizona Cardinals a few weeks after he entered free agency and decided to leave the Texans. During his first press conference in Arizona, he spoke in a measured cadence as he respectfully answered all the reporters' questions and said how pleased he was to join the team, the city, and its fans. Then a reporter asked about his relationship with his new teammates. JJ's voice quickened and rose a few decibels as he leaned forward in his chair:

> *I can't wait to get out there and work with [my teammates], just put in the work, be on the practice field talking about schemes we want to run together...how we see things... that's one of the most fun parts of the game is when you have guys who love the game, and love studying film, and love being on the practice field, and love putting in the work. When you have a full team of guys like that who have a passion for winning and have a drive for wanting to be great. That's when football's just the best, because then you feed off of each other....*

JJ did not speak of the money he would make, the fame he would gain, or the championships he would win. Instead, he spoke of the meaningful connections he would share with teammates in pursuit of a common dream and the hard work it would take to attain that dream.

A person with cancer suffers from a terrifying disease that will probably take his life and maybe even steal much of his humanity, but cancer is not his whole life. He has lived this amazing life with all those passions that cancer can never take away. The spark that brings life to those passions is love: love between patients and those who care for them, love between family members who lay down their mobile phones long enough to create a quilt together, and love between a football player and his teammates. Life indeed imitates art, but the art of medicine imitates the lives of people who clinicians are fortunate enough to meet along the way.

PRACTICE POINTS

Key Reflections

- The best way to imagine what a person is thinking or feeling is to ask him to tell you about his life—his passions, accomplishments, hopes, fears, and dreams—and then to listen carefully. This is the essential first step in empathic practice.

- Oscar Wilde said, "Life imitates Art." However, for empathic clinicians, the art of medicine sometimes imitates life.

- Empathy need not be reserved only for difficult conversations about goals of care, prognosis, and other sensitive topics. Clinicians can weave empathy into the fabric of every encounter by speaking about everyday topics rather than just about medical issues. This can be thought of as speaking to patients like people rather than just as patients.

- Speaking to patients about everyday topics usually takes only a few minutes and is time well spent on strengthening our connections to them.

- A person's legacy is arguably much more valuable than traditional measures of success, such as fame, fortune, and power.

- A person with cancer suffers from a terrifying disease that will probably take his life and maybe even steal much of his humanity, but cancer is not his whole life. He has lived this amazing life with all those passions that cancer can never take away.

Empathic Actions

- Occasionally introducing humor into clinical encounters can be healing by offering patients moments of reprieve from the weight of their illness and allowing them to live in the moment.

- The most effective humor respects the patient, follows their verbal and nonverbal cues, and focuses on universal human themes.

- Respecting a patient's religious faith, love of family, resilience, fighting spirit, legacy, and other meaningful personal attributes is deeply empathic.

Empathic Expression

- "Please, no need to apologize about asking questions. I can see how much you love him."

- "You are doing an amazing job caring for him. I respect how you always advocate for your husband. I also think that both of you have done a great job raising your children, based on what I know about them. Raising nice children is no small feat."

- "You may be lucky to have such wonderful children, but I think you have also set a great example and have raised them right. Your role as parents and grandparents is arguably the most important part of your legacy."

- "From what I can tell from prior conversations, you also treat your employees like family, so you can feel confident that your legacy is secure, regardless of how long you live."

14 Data Synthesis in the Pursuit of Personhood

Donna S. Zhukovsky and Daniel E. Epner

REFLECTING ON WHAT is it to be an empathic clinician, I recalled a patient who touched my heart when I saw her as a consultation with one of the nurse practitioners on our team. Ms. R was a single woman in her early 30s who had progressive metastatic rectal cancer complicated by a large pelvic fluid collection, a malfunctioning pelvic drain, and poorly controlled pain despite the use of high doses of opioids. Adding to the complexity of her situation, she had survived three cardiac arrests over the past few weeks. Before meeting Ms. R, my colleague and I discussed her at length, during which time the nurse practitioner presented a comprehensive data review that included results of the Edmonton Symptom Assessment Scale, the Memorial Delirium Assessment Scale, the patient's family structure and job history, pain medication history, morphine equivalent daily dose, physical findings, and imaging results. She also described how our team had rotated the patient's opioid regimen multiple times, never finding a regimen that provided Ms. R with adequate relief. The nurse practitioner did an excellent job of collecting and presenting objective data for us to consider as we developed a treatment plan.

Pain Perception Is Complex

Among our concerns was that this young woman seemed to require higher doses of opioids every day, particularly in the intravenous form, than we expected based on imaging findings, physical exam, and our subjective assessment of her comfort and function. She appeared to be comfortable taking a few steps in her room or walking short distances around the nursing unit; however, she often became very demonstrative about her pain in our team's presence. Considering the patient's pelvic collection to be the source of her pain, the nurse practitioner suggested that we ask interventional radiology to reposition the malfunctioning drain, potentially a much more effective intervention than increasing opioids if the undrained tumor abscess was the source of her pain. However, the longer we discussed the situation, the more it became clear to me that we would have to do much more than reposition the drain to address this woman's pain. Going through her chart more thoroughly, I learned that she had a past psychiatric history that related to unspecified teenage trauma, with the possibility that earlier emotional, physical, and/or sexual abuse could be contributing to her current pain experience. This woman's pain was not just bodily pain, but rather a deeper suffering that opioids and other medications could not fully relieve.

Synthesizing the Data

Thinking about Ms. R, I realize that we clinicians are often under excruciating time pressure, and consequently become focused on completing our assessments and checking off our to-do lists rather than stepping back, reflecting on the information coming at us in real time, and looking at the patient as a person. I like to refer to this reflective process as "synthesizing" the data, which can be thought of as combining many facts into a coherent whole, or said otherwise, putting the pieces of the puzzle together. This type of synthesis requires slowing down long enough to imagine what the patient and family are thinking and feeling, which is the essence of empathy. Of course, everyone does this in his or her own unique way, but success depends on weaving the many pieces of the medical and psychosocial histories into a cohesive story in a natural and free-flowing way. This is especially important when pieces of the picture don't add up. Part of this synthesis extends beyond chart review to a reciprocal process whereby the clinician tunes into the patient's and family's words and nonverbal communication and adapts to the resulting sensory input, rather than imposing an agenda on the patient. This adaptive process allows patients to express themselves fully and thereby builds trust and rapport, yielding a deeper level of understanding.

Addressing Existential Distress

After introducing myself to the young woman, her mother, and her aunt, the first thing I asked was, "What's your biggest worry?" She replied, "I am worried my pain will get so bad that I will have to get around in a wheelchair." Given her debility and the progressive nature of her cancer, I could not reassure her that this would not become her reality, so I replied, "Using a wheelchair would be a huge change for you, since you were so independent and active before your illness. Tell me more about what worries you most about using a wheelchair." She explained that she left an abusive and chaotic home when she was just a teenager and had two children at a young age, but that her children's father was no longer in the picture. Close friends had agreed to care for her children during hospital stays, but she knew they would not be available long-term, so she worried about her children's future. She had many reasons to be terrified in addition to incurable cancer. The more I listened, the more I connected with her, and the more I connected, the more I realized this woman was experiencing tremendous existential distress. According to Eric Cassell's writings, her sense of self was threatened.

After listening silently for several minutes, I said, "I can only imagine what you are going through. I can tell how much you love your children." I then asked her what she liked to do when she was not feeling sick. It turned out that she loved creating art. To build on restoring her sense of self, I asked her family to bring in some small art projects, as her energy was limited and I did not want to overwhelm her. She did not seem very enthusiastic about this idea, so I asked her what other things she enjoyed doing. She talked about how much she liked the music scene and being with her friends, so I asked if she was keeping in touch with her friends by FaceTime. Then she changed the subject and started telling me how much she loved her horses and wanted nothing more than to hang out in the barn with them to brush their coats and manes, feed them, give them sponge baths, and change their bedding. As she daydreamed about her horses, she gazed into the distance as if imagining the sensation of running her hands gently over one of her horse's velvety noses while smelling the earthy fragrance of hay, oats, and manure. She then told me about her two dogs and a cat, and I said, "Well, I don't know if it's possible to bring a pet here now because of the coronavirus pandemic, but we have a program that sometimes arranges for people to bring their dogs to the hospital. We can look into it." At that point, her face lit up with a huge smile as she quickly suggested that her cousin might be able to help her mom bring her dog to the hospital for a visit. I then told her how much I could relate to her enthusiasm because I, too, find spending time with my dog Lucy to be comforting and a source of joy. Mentioning Lucy was not idle chitchat but rather what many call "therapeutic use of self," which is giving the patient a glimpse of our life in order to connect on the human level and solidify our relationship.

Discussing her love of animals and particularly her dog was my first big win, even though we had not yet arranged a visit. She was excited that I discussed the possibility of a pet visit through the PAWS program (Pets Are Wonderful Support, https://www.pawshouston.org/). We then talked about other integrative concepts, such as music therapy, massage, acupuncture, and other mind-body interventions, for which she seemed very grateful. We arranged for our clinical psychologist to see her and discussed strategies for allowing her children to visit. I think I was able to connect with her by putting discussion of medical topics like medications and symptoms to the side for a few minutes while focusing on her humanity.

Giving the Patient as Much Control as Possible

I then returned to medical issues by briefly summarizing my conversation with the nurse practitioner rather than making the patient repeat everything from scratch, which showed my respect for both the patient and my colleague. I asked her to tell me a little bit more about the pain, letting her describe it in her own words for a few minutes, and said, "I hear that you got a better response from drug X than you did from drug Y." We then discussed the various options for medication regimens and doses, potential side effects, and safety issues. We negotiated as she asked several questions and stated her preferences, but in the final analysis, she chose her preferred regimen from the medically appropriate options I presented to her. In other words, she owned the final plan rather than having to agree reluctantly to one that I recommended and thereby derived a sense of control over at least one aspect of her life. This represented another small victory, since she had so little control over anything else. For days leading up to our meeting, this young woman had insisted on using intravenous pain medicines excessively and had been very demanding toward nursing staff, but after our discussion about art, integrative medicine, dogs, and her beloved horses, she and her family accepted my recommendation and her interactions with the staff became much calmer. We also ended up adjusting her pelvic drain, as originally suggested by the nurse practitioner. As we left the room with our plan in place, the patient, her mother, and her aunt exuded a palpable sense of relief. They felt that we viewed her as more than a patient with cancer and a malfunctioning abscess drain, but rather as a person with a rich lifetime of experiences. Her previous high pain expression was a cry for help, reflecting existential distress rather than a malfunctioning drain. We subsequently transferred her to the acute palliative care unit for further symptom management. Five days later, after receiving counseling on how to best support each of her young children, she returned home with hospice care to spend quality time with her children and family.

PRACTICE POINTS

Key Reflections

- Caring for patients effectively and compassionately requires "synthesizing" voluminous biomedical data, which can be thought of as combining many facts into a coherent whole or putting the pieces of the puzzle together.

- Synthesizing biomedical data requires slowing down long enough to imagine what the patient and family are thinking and feeling, which is the essence of empathy.

- Pain perception is highly subjective and heavily influenced by many factors other than tissue injury.

- Pain is a complex construct accentuated by negative emotions, such as fear and anxiety.

- A significant proportion of patients with ready access to opioids, particularly in the IV form, take them for reasons other than pain, such as to alleviate anxiety. Many pain management experts refer to this phenomenon as "chemical coping" or high pain expression.

- "Therapeutic use of self" is the process of giving a patient a glimpse into our personal lives in order to connect on the human level while not distracting from the patient's needs.

Empathic Actions

- Discussing nonmedical issues and facilitating access to integrative resources, such as music therapy, massage, acupuncture, and pets, respects the patient's humanity and dignity.

- Strategic use of medical procedures, such as insertion or replacement of drains and catheters, can have great palliative benefit even for patients who are approaching the end of life.

Empathic Expression

- Open-ended questions, such as "What is your biggest worry?" or "What do you hope for?," allow patients to express their emotions and thereby create empathic opportunities.

- Patient: *I am worried my pain will get so bad that I will have to get around in a wheelchair.*

- Traditional response:

  - *Do not give up hope. I think we can get you strong enough to be able to walk again.*

- ○ Recommended empathic response:

  - ▪ *Using a wheelchair would be a huge change for you, since you were so independent and active before your illness. Tell me more about what worries you most about using a wheelchair.*

  - ▪ Patient replies: *I am worried I won't be able to care for my children if I am stuck in a wheelchair.*

  - ▪ *That must be a scary thought. I can tell how much you want the best for your children.*

- • Patient: *I am worried no one will take care of my children after I die.*

  - ○ Traditional response:

    - ▪ *Do you have parents, siblings, or other family members who can take over for you?*

  - ○ Recommended empathic response:

    - ▪ *I can only imagine what you are going through. I can tell how much you love your children.*

15 | The Backstory Is Really the Front Story

Shiao-Pei Weathers and Daniel E. Epner

EMANUEL KANT, THE 18th-century German philosopher, said, "We can judge the heart of a man by his treatment of animals." If so, my maternal grandfather must have had a kind and generous heart, since he rescued stray Pariah dogs from the streets of Mumbai, India and welcomed them into his family. I recently came across a sepia-toned picture of my grandfather as a young man in one of our family photo albums. In the photo, he smiled broadly as he cradled a brown and white Pariah puppy, supporting the dog's soft underbelly with one arm and stroking him between the ears with the other. That puppy was only one of a long line of lucky canines who found refuge and love in his house. As the youngest of five children, my mother helped bathe, feed, and play with the dogs, who served as her constant companions throughout childhood. Dogs have been an integral part of our family for over four generations.

Both my parents' families are ethnically Chinese, from Hubei Province. However, when Communists took over China after the Second World War, my grandparents fled by the most direct route available to them, which was to India, where both of my parents were born. Other Chinese professionals fled to Pakistan, Afghanistan, or other neighboring countries. The Chinese community in India during the 1960s and '70s was quite small and tight-knit. As a result, my dad's parents in Calcutta knew my mom's parents in Mumbai, even though the two cities are separated by almost 1300 miles. When my dad traveled to and from his home in Calcutta to the United States during his psychiatry residency, he had to pass through Mumbai, India's major commercial center, where he stayed with my mom's family and met her during those brief layovers. My parents must have been very compatible, because they married after a brief courtship that consisted primarily of corresponding by letter, and they remain happily married many years later. When my dad landed a permanent position in the United States in Kentucky, he sponsored my mom to join him. They had to quickly assimilate into American culture in Kentucky, since so few Chinese people lived there.

When I grew up in Kentucky for the first nine years of my life and subsequently in a rural town in Ohio, all my friends had dogs. Having a dog seemed quintessentially American, so I wanted one too. However, my parents were strict, and I was an only child, so they insisted that I prove that I could care for a dog. My parents' greatest fear was that my love of dogs would be a passing fad and that they would be stuck taking care of a family dog if we got one. Fortunately, we had neighbors who had two Yorkshire Terriers who I would dog sit when I was 13 to prove I could and would bathe them, feed them, walk them, and groom them. After a few years of dog sitting, I earned my parents' trust and we got Tiffany, a Yorkie, the same breed I had cared for at my neighbor's house. Tiffany lived for almost 14 years, until after I graduated from medical school. I was too busy to care for her when I left for college and even after I returned to live at home during medical school, but by that time, my mother had developed a strong relationship with Tiffany and was delighted to care for her as she had the many dogs of her youth. Tiffany reciprocated by serving as a loyal source of emotional support for my mom when she received treatment for breast cancer at a time when my dad and I were busy with our careers. Tiffany loved my mom unconditionally, even after her hair fell out and she lost weight during chemotherapy. Tiffany seemed to know that my mom was sick and responded by lavishing her with even more love and attention.

The Queen of the Backstory

My love of dogs has helped me connect with patients in my neuro-oncology practice. One of my main goals has always been to learn something personal about my patients beyond their medical history and basic social history. This may sound cheesy, but if something is important to my patient, it should be important to me. For instance, I try to remember details like how many children a patient has, their names, ages, birthdays, and special hobbies. I try to go beyond information that most people discuss in clinic to establish an ongoing dialogue from visit to visit. For instance, I may say, "I remember you were going to take a trip to Ireland. How was it? Do you have pictures?" Every time a fellow works with me in clinic, I try to set a good example by mentioning some personal detail about a patient that I gleaned during a previous visit. However, I often find myself disappointed by the fellows' lack of enthusiasm about these details. Then I recall my own years of training and remind myself that learners are forced to assimilate enormous amounts of biomedical knowledge in order to gain basic proficiency in neuro-oncology, so it often takes them several years to fully appreciate the human side of medicine. One of my colleagues, a neurosurgeon, recently called me the "queen of the backstory" based on my focus on patients' personal lives. However, information that others dub the backstory is the glue that helps me connect with patients and most effectively guide them through the uncertainties and fear associated with cancer and its treatment. People's illnesses should not define them. Maybe we should think of the tumor as the backstory and the violin, woodshop, or family pet as the front story.

Sometimes remembering a patient's personal details can be a double-edged sword, because I become more attached to them and find it more difficult to separate work from home. I also grieve more when I share disappointing news, which is unavoidable for patients with brain tumors. For me, suffering is not an abstract concept. When I see patients in the clinic, they present their best selves to me, but I often imagine what their lives must be like at home away from my view. I envision them stumbling over stairs and curbs, grasping for words, and losing control of basic bodily functions as cancer steals their dignity. How sad and frustrating must it be for a patient to no longer be able to tell his son or daughter "I love you"? How humiliating must it be for an adult to need help toileting? I often ruminate about patients all weekend since I see them in clinic on Friday. Nonetheless, the joy I feel from bonding with my patients meaningfully more than makes up for the sadness I feel when they lose their power and autonomy and ultimately die. I am still relatively early in my career, so I hope over time I will be able to maintain this balance and avoid burnout.

Connecting with a Patient Through Our Mutual Love of Dogs

Mrs. G was a 63-year-old woman with glioblastoma, the most lethal form of brain cancer. She recovered well from surgery and traveled to my clinic to discuss chemotherapy, which we planned to combine with radiation. She was still independent the first time I met her and presented to clinic alone. While I was pleased by her mobility, I was concerned by her apparent social isolation. Her physical appearance spoke of a hard life.

Her cutoff jeans hung baggily around her spindly legs, suggesting a lifetime of poor nutrition. Bruises and abrasions covered her fragile, sun-damaged skin. She often wore tattered souvenir T-shirts from early '90s rock concerts, and her hair was unruly. When I first met her, she was polite but subdued, seemed wary of my intentions, and was slightly tremulous. I introduced myself briefly and then immediately said, "You seem worried. What's on your mind?" Her eyes met mine momentarily, and then she quickly gazed down at her lap while laughing faintly, waved her hand dismissively, and said, "Oh nothing, I'm fine." She seemed like a secret diary, locked tight against prying eyes. I changed to a safer topic, namely informed consent, side effects, and logistics of chemotherapy, and we continued to speak primarily about medical issues for the first few visits.

After a while, we fell into the familiar rhythm of chemotherapy every few weeks alternating with clinic checkups. During these routine visits, I gradually learned more about her life and discovered that her husband committed suicide. After her husband's death but before her cancer diagnosis, Mrs. G. became even more socially isolated and contemplated suicide, but she decided against it after seeing the devastating effect that her husband's suicide had on their only daughter. I also learned from conversations with her primary care provider that she battled depression for many years before her cancer diagnosis. Our increasingly personal conversations not only provided valuable information about how I could best care for her in the context of her complex psychosocial situation, but more importantly gradually built trust between us.

I soon learned that Mrs. G loved dogs as much as I do. She lived alone on a large plot of land in the country where she worked as a home health aide. She was so isolated that the closest grocery store was a 40-minute drive. As a result, she always kept a German shepherd for security as well as two Pomeranians, JoJo and NuNu. Mrs. G came to life when she spoke of her dogs. The first time I mentioned dogs, Mrs. G looked up from her lap with tears welling in her eyes and described how she had fostered seven Pomeranians at one point and had helped place several of them into stable homes. Her voice rose with excitement whenever she described her "baby" JoJo, a Pomeranian that she specifically bought for herself and raised since she was a puppy. As she spoke, I reached for my phone to show her pictures of our family dog, Cocoa, a Shih Tzu-Bichon mix (Shichon), frolicking with our daughter, Olivia, in the yard. Olivia and Cocoa wore matching red and green sweaters as they chased each other and dispersed a pile of leaves my husband had just raked. Mrs. G gazed longingly at the photos, imagining such a life, mourning many lost opportunities with her daughter, Trudy, wondering where she went wrong and why all the important people in her life had abandoned her. She tried whenever possible to forget her illness by shoving it into the dark recesses of her mind, but when she traveled to clinic for appointments she was forced to face it in the light of day. She wished dearly that she could cradle JoJo in her arms during those visits. JoJo was Mrs. G's sole source of meaning and was a surrogate daughter to replace Trudy, who was addicted to drugs, was unfailingly attracted to abusive men, and was constantly in trouble with the law. However, Trudy could be charming at times as a way of manipulating Mrs. G and stealing money from her to support her drug habit. Child protective services eventually deemed Trudy unfit as a parent and took custody of her daughter, another setback in a seemingly endless cycle of familial suffering and despair. The final straw was when Ms. G concluded that Trudy broke into her home, stole NuNu, and sold the dog to support her drug habit, although Mrs. G could never prove it. After that, Mrs. G. severed ties with Trudy forever and clung to JoJo as tightly as she clung to her own life.

One day Mrs. G arrived in clinic appearing more distressed than usual and seemed distracted and disengaged. When I looked at her inquisitively, she volunteered that her German shepherd had a seizure recently in her kitchen and died suddenly. The story never made sense to me, but the way Ms. G. told it, she was too weak to carry the dog's remains, so she decided to drag it out to the yard for burial. However, the dog entered rigor mortis, so Mrs. G was forced to break all the dog's legs post mortem to fit her in a large plastic trash bag. I became slightly nauseated as I imagined my patient breaking her dog into pieces like a dead branch. I was struck by how Ms. G's life seemed like an old Western movie in which settlers lived in isolation, fended for themselves, huddled together against the cold in rough-hewn cabins, and nearly starved during long, snowy winters. In those days, tiny mounds of dirt dotted family cemetery plots as grim reminders of the many babies and toddlers who died suddenly from illness or exposure. As disturbed as I was by Mrs. G's story, I was even more disturbed by the way that she told it. She never shed a tear and described the scene matter-of-factly, almost robotically. She seemed to push through the trauma and chaos in her life as if in a trance, floating outside her body while seeing her pain, fear, and anxiety as abstractions. How could her soul hurt if it was already hollow and dead, like a rotten tree branch? She came to believe that she was not worthy of any person's love, including her own. She must have reasoned that her constant companion and protector, her beloved German shepherd, was dead anyway, so she could not feel pain while being dismembered and stuffed into a plastic bag. Besides, Mrs. G knew her dog's soul was bound for heaven, even though she dared not imagine where her own soul was headed. As I listened to Mrs. G's story, I felt a mixture of admiration, revulsion, and pathos. Mrs. G's beloved NuNu was gone to points unknown, presumably taken by her daughter, and her German shepherd was buried in the backyard. JoJo was all that remained, and Mrs. G. needed JoJo's love like she needed air.

An Unusual Request

After a few months, Ms. G's tumor grew as expected, and as a result, she became increasingly debilitated and began to neglect herself even more. I soon asked our social worker to contact

Adult Protective Services (APS), who inspected Mrs. G's home and concurred that she was unable to live alone safely. With the help of APS, we established a power of attorney for Ms. G, a retired nurse named Josephine who Ms. G met many years ago when she helped care for Josephine's mother after a stroke. Josephine was a breath of fresh air whose boundless energy and positivity breathed life into Ms. G's world. Before Mrs. G lost the ability to communicate, Josephine and I met with her to discuss various safe places for her to live. I started the conversation. "Mrs. G, I am concerned this is as strong as you will get. I do not think you can care for yourself any longer." I let this profound news sink in, because I was sure Mrs. G would resist moving from her land in the country. However, she seemed resigned to the fact that she could no longer go it alone. She continued to stare at her lap for a few seconds and then nodded her head in agreement. She then started to weep silently and asked, "What about JoJo?" Josephine and I looked at each other, realizing that we had not considered the most important question. None of the facilities that Josephine had identified accepted dogs. Mrs. G continued, "I know I can't live by myself, but I need to live somewhere that will let JoJo live with me. I can't live without JoJo." I was proud of myself and our team for having taken the initiative to address Mrs. G's psychosocial needs, but I began to feel slightly embarrassed for having not considered JoJo. Josephine and I sat in silence thinking about what to say. After several seconds, Mrs. G continued: "I suppose I could live somewhere without JoJo and meet my maker in peace as long as I know she will be well taken care of in a loving home. I want JoJo to live in a home full of life, because I haven't been able to take care of her the way I wanted these past few months." Toward the end of her life, Ms. G became so debilitated that she had trouble getting up to feed JoJo, let alone bathe her or take her to the vet. As she spoke, I envisioned my daughter Olivia holding our dog Cocoa in her lap on the couch at home. Mrs. G turned to me, inhaled deeply to summon her courage, and said, "I trust you. Will you take JoJo?" I thought I misunderstood her. Did my patient just ask me to adopt her dog? Her question both flattered and disarmed me. I had clearly succeeded in connecting with Mrs. G on a deeply human level, but I also feared that I had torn down an invisible shield that we doctors so often build to protect ourselves from the intense fires of grief. Maybe my colleague was right when he jokingly referred to me as the queen of the backstory. Stalling for time, I told Mrs. G I would ask my husband and let her know as soon as possible.

Rebirth

I knew my husband, Bret, would not stand in the way of adopting Jojo, far from it. In fact, I knew he would be delighted to adopt another dog, but I needed time to decide whether I was comfortable with the arrangement. When Bret and I first met during medical school in Ohio, I could tell a lot about him by the way he treated his mom. He called his mom every day, even if it was just to say, "I'm doing okay, got a test next week but everything is fine. I love you." He may have only spoken to her for 30 seconds or a minute, but he knew how much those calls meant to her. Bret also grew up in a very observant Christian home, and he lives by Christian ideals. He has always looked out for the little guy and is never motivated by personal recognition. When he was in high school, he was the only popular and accomplished boy in his class who befriended kids who others considered "geeky" or "nerdy" and defended them against bullies. He also loves animals as much as he loves people. Ironically, I often think Brett should have been a veterinarian rather than a doctor, because he always tells me that his dream job is to have acres and acres of land so that he can adopt all the dogs without a home and give them a big place to live. His family always had a dog from the time he was a baby growing up in Kansas. So, I met zero resistance from Bret when I asked him whether we could adopt JoJo. He was more than happy to provide Olivia and Cocoa another playmate, but the real question was whether I would be comfortable crossing into what seemed like forbidden territory for medical professionals. After giving the matter serious consideration, I decided that adopting JoJo was the right thing to do.

One week later, Bret and I loaded Olivia and Cocoa in the car on Sunday after church and drove two hours into the countryside to meet Mrs. G at a McDonald's in her small Texas town. She waited for us in the parking lot while holding JoJo in her arms, flanked by the friend who drove her there. She quickly sized up my family as we walked toward her and then summoned all her strength to hold JoJo at chest level and enthusiastically announce, "This is my little JoJo! What do you think?" Then, without waiting for a reply, she handed JoJo over to me as she looked down at JoJo and said, "I know you will be so happy with your new friends Cocoa and Olivia. You are going to have a wonderful time." There was no turning back for either of us. As we parted ways, Mrs. G looked like the mother on a sinking ship who had just placed her young child in the one remaining seat in the lifeboat.

JoJo seemed disoriented during that initial car trip back to Houston and panted with anxiety the whole way. In fact, she slept and ate poorly for the first few weeks in her new surroundings. We took her to the vet three days after we adopted her for an exam and blood work that revealed poor nutrition, hypothyroidism, poor dentition, and hair loss. We spent $850 on dental care to treat several rotten teeth that undoubtedly hurt, and after a few weeks, she gained weight and grew a full shiny coat. Before long, she even started following me around like a shadow with what appeared to be a smile on her face. At first, she slept with me every night, but after a few weeks, she started sleeping in her bed on her back, tummy up, which is a vulnerable position and the true sign of a secure and happy dog. Now, we always take her on car rides with Cocoa and treat them like sisters, with matching collars and personalized beds, and we include her in all our holiday and birthday photos. Cocoa and JoJo participate in the normal sibling rivalry, a sure sign that JoJo has become one of the gang.

A Resting Place for Mrs. G

I saw Mrs. G in clinic a few more times after we adopted JoJo, and each time I shared several photos of JoJo in her new life. In one photo she posed proudly with a pink bow in her hair after a bath and blow-dry. In another she sat between Olivia and Cocoa securely strapped into the back seat of our car on a drive in the country. Mrs. G. no longer grieved. Instead, she appeared as though she had finally found peace. Examining her life, she had many regrets, but she finally felt secure in the knowledge that she definitely did one thing right. She found JoJo a seat in the lifeboat.

Once JoJo was secure, we turned our full attention to finding a place for Mrs. G to live out her final days in comfort. We initially thought she should live in a skilled nursing facility, but we could not find one that would accept her health insurance. Then, as we deliberated during one of her last visits, Mrs. G suddenly said, "Maybe I can live in Topeka." Josephine and I looked at each other in stunned silence and then asked, "Why Topeka?" I had spent many hours caring for Mrs. G and had learned much about her life, but until that moment I had no idea that she grew up in Topeka, Kansas and still had a sister and several childhood friends there. Understanding how chaotic and solitary Mrs. G's life had become, I doubted her sister would have anything to do with her. However, to my surprise, I soon learned that her sister was delighted to welcome her back into the family. In fact, she drove all the way from Topeka to Houston to pick her up. After a life filled with sorrow, anger, and fear, Mrs. G found comfort in the company of friends and family and died peacefully 2 months after we adopted JoJo.

In Christianity, we often speak of Heaven as a place of infinite beauty and peace, where deserving souls live in bliss forever. However, Heaven remains a mystery to me, a place I cannot envision as hard as I try. Maybe Heaven is not a destination as we think but rather a mysterious network of souls whirling around the Universe, touching, reshaping, and redirecting all other souls, both living and dead, much like neurons and neurotransmitters reshape networks in the brain. Tumors can steal a woman's physical prowess and life, but her soul remains. I like to think that Mrs. G's soul lives within JoJo, me, and my family, bathed in the love and tranquility of our home. Mrs. G helped me see that there are no backstories or front stories. I now know that there are only human stories, of tragedy and triumph, of sorrow and joy, and of fear and security. The most powerful stories are stories of love, always imperfect but nonetheless transcendent; love between mothers and their daughters, love between people and animals, and love between doctors and their patients: stories that live on in all of us forever.

PRACTICE POINTS

Key Reflections

- Clinicians connect most meaningfully with their patients when they learn about their humanity and important aspects of their personal lives in addition to attending to their medical issues.

- If something is important to a patient, it should be important to the clinicians caring for that patient.

- Clinicians can heal patients by helping them live as well as possible even when they cannot cure their disease.

- Trainees in complex medical fields spend so much time and effort acquiring technical knowledge and skills that they often need years of practice before they can fully appreciate the human side and art of medicine.

- Clinicians who form strong bonds with patients run the risk of experiencing heightened grief when their patients suffer. Nonetheless, the joy resulting from those close bonds can more than compensate for the sadness of witnessing suffering and death.

- An astute clinician can often tell a lot about a patient's life experiences, mental health, and emotional well-being at first glance, much like a good detective can often solve a crime by examining a crime scene carefully.

- Mental illness, physical and mental abuse, and neglect are common aspects of patients' psychosocial histories that greatly impact clinicians' ability to care for them.

Empathic Actions

- Medical practice is a team sport. The best clinicians are those who involve social workers, counselors, adult protective services, child protective services, and other non-clinicians to help them address their patients' most vexing psychosocial issues.

- Patients are most likely to trust clinicians who connect with them on a human level.

- Trust is required for clinicians and their patients to create therapeutic alliance.

- Clinicians who form strong trusting relationships with their patients are more likely to cope well with stressors inherent in caring for seriously ill patients.

- Clinicians who wish to go above and beyond traditional clinical roles in order to establish therapeutic alliance with their patients should still maintain proper professional boundaries and objectivity.

Empathic Expression

- (Exploration) "You seem worried. What is on your mind?"

- "I remember you were going to take a trip to Ireland. How was it? Do you have pictures?"

- "I am concerned this is as strong as you will get. I do not think you can care for yourself any longer."

- "I wish we had better treatment options for you."

16 | The Angel on My Shoulder

Michael Frumovitz and Daniel E. Epner

My PATIENT WAS a 36-year-old woman with recurrent small cell carcinoma of the cervix, an incurable condition. In addition to facing the prospect of death, she also faced the collateral damage that cancer invariably inflicts on its victims' personal lives. "Who will care for my children?" she asked through sobs. "My husband can't be trusted. He's a no-good drunk and a cheat who can't hold down a job. My parents are divorced and my mother has a bad heart." Then after a brief pause to consider her seemingly hopeless circumstances, she steeled her resolve and said, "I'm not giving up! I have to be here for my children." It was late in the afternoon, at the end of a clinic packed with many other patients who faced similarly grave prognoses. I operated that morning from 6:30 until clinic began at noon, so I was fried and desperately needed to finish my work and get home. Yet her plaintive voice droned on, and as it did, the proverbial angel on my shoulder engaged in mortal combat with the devil on my other shoulder. The little angel stood tall and proud as always in his starched white coat, clean-shaven and composed. He said, "Stay calm. Take a breath. Stick with it. Give her a few more minutes." However, her sobbing showed no signs of abating, so the little devil emerged from his cave and crawled up on my shoulder wearing dirty scrubs and a three-day beard, disheveled, frustrated, and exhausted. He yelled in my ear, "I can't take another minute of this. I need to get out of here before I scream! What does she expect me to do or say about her personal problems?" As I thought about how to respond, I wondered, "What would Dad do in this situation?"

A Major Role Model

My dad was an obstetrician-gynecologist in private practice in Santa Monica, California. He spent most of his life in New York and then spent the first two years of his career after residency at Edwards Air Force base in the Mojave Desert caring for the wives of service members during the Vietnam War. After his military service, family beckoned from the north, but the allure of sunny California was too strong. Although his practice was in Santa Monica, my parents could not afford a house there, so they built one in Malibu, which was about 15-minutes' drive from the hospital. This was the '70s, a time when Malibu was still a beach community rather than the playground of the rich and famous it is today. I remember many trailer parks up and down Pacific Coast Highway, although we lived in a regular, middle-class neighborhood. Nonetheless, my dad cared for several famous actors who lived near his office in Santa Monica. One day, my father asked one of his new patients what she did for work, as he did all his patients. When this young woman replied that she was an actor, my dad asked, "What restaurant do you work in?" since nearly all young actors worked in bars and restaurants to pay the bills until they could get steady acting jobs. When she explained that she did not work in a restaurant, he asked again, "No, really, what restaurant do you work in?" Slightly amused at that point, she replied, "I used to work in restaurants, but I am past that now. In fact, I appeared in two movies this year." "Oh, really? Which movies?" he asked. She named the two films, both of which were huge box office hits in which she starred alongside several Hollywood luminaries. This woman was no bit player, so I think my dad was one of few people in the world who did not know her. He then replied without a trace of embarrassment, "Oh, I haven't seen those yet. I will make a point of seeing them as soon as I get a chance." As it turns out, he never saw either movie. He had no interest in fawning over his patients or seeking favors or recognition, which is one of the many reasons why his patients trusted and respected him so much. When my dad was not spending time with my mother, my brothers, and me, he focused exclusively on providing his patients the best care possible, regardless of whether they were homemakers, homeless people, or Hollywood luminaries. On another occasion, he met one of his patients at a sporting event accompanied by her husband. She is also an actor whose husband is one of the most famous and decorated actors in recent decades. When they spotted my dad from a distance, both immediately jostled their way through the crowd just to get access to my dad, shake his hand, and tell him how happy they were to see him. Perhaps for the first time in their lives, my dad's patient and her husband were the paparazzi. Naturally, this encounter left my dad mortified, since the last thing he sought was limelight. Another of my dad's famous patients called the clinic the day before her appointment to insist that the staff clear the waiting room before she arrived to ensure her privacy. When his staff approached him with the request, he quietly declined. She showed up and waited (briefly) like everyone else. He treated all his patients the same, which is to say like royalty.

Besides treating all his patients the same regardless of their social status, my dad also constantly demonstrated how deeply he cared for them. I remember many nights when I was in high school when I would return from a party or school function at midnight or 2 am and see my dad wearing out the carpet in his study, pacing the floor as he contemplated how he would help a patient who was experiencing a rough postoperative course. He could barely wait for the clock to strike five, when he could return to the hospital to turn things around. I also remember many occasions when I was 8 or 10 when my dad would pick my younger brother and me up from school and make a quick house call on the way home to check on one of his patients. He would leave my brother and me in the car for the few minutes he spent in the house, and then reward us with ice cream or another treat on the final leg of our trip home. This practice seemed routine to me at the time. However, it was not until I began my medical training in the 1990s that I appreciated that house calls were very special in that era, several decades after small town country doctors traveled back roads carrying their black bags. On other occasions, he took us with him to the hospital when he made brief rounds on weekends even though he was not on call. He plopped us down in the cafeteria and told us we could eat whatever we wanted while he checked on his patients. In these ways, my brother and I danced around the fringes of my dad's clinical practice, but we never actually saw him interact with patients in the clinical setting. Nonetheless, we could tell how deeply he cared about his patients just by watching him from a distance. My father embodied Francis Peabody's famous quote: "The secret of the care of the patient is in caring for the patient."

Focusing on a Rare and Often Lethal Cancer

My father was a community obstetrician-gynecologist, but I decided to pursue an academic career as a gynecological oncologist. When I started my academic career, I did not consciously choose to focus my research and clinical work on small cell carcinoma of the cervix, which is a rare entity. My career path evolved in unpredictable ways as it does for many people. When I first joined the faculty at MD Anderson Cancer Center in the early 2000s, one of my senior colleagues received funding for a clinical trial sponsored by a pharmaceutical company that studied the possible role of bevacizumab for treating small cell cervical cancer. He handed the trial over to me to get me started in research. The problem was that we only enrolled about three patients in the first two years, because we did not have the same network to recruit patients as we have now. As a result, the company closed the study. A few years later, a group of women with small cell cervical cancer found each other on Facebook and formed a support group, because they had this sense of isolation due to the rareness of their cancer. About a year into it, about 20 or 30 women participated in this group, and they decided to raise money for research. Then they had to find some research to fund. None of the original group knew me, but they must have searched the internet for research trials for their condition and my name was the only one that surfaced based on our unsuccessful clinical trial. They approached me and told me about their plan to fund research, and I asked what kind of research they wanted to fund. They told me they wanted to establish a full translational research program with lab studies and clinical trials, which sounded to me like a $2 million research program. I enthusiastically told them I was all in and asked how much money they thought they could raise. When they replied $25–30,000, we discussed a more focused initial strategy. I said, "Why don't we start with something easy like an informational website, because nothing exists yet for patient and clinician education." Then, we used the website as a portal through which we recruited into our tumor registry to get an idea of the natural history of the disease and prognosis. This was over 10 years ago, so very little information was available. Since we started the small cell cervical cancer website, the Facebook group has expanded dramatically and now has hundreds of members.

Small cell cervical cancer, a subtype of high-grade neuroen-docrine carcinoma, often affects women in their 20s or early 30s. Caring for young patients who sometimes have children of their own as well as parents who are involved in their care can be very emotionally challenging, especially for the nurse practitioners in our department, many of whom are young women who naturally identify with our patients. The stakes are very high. Sixty per-cent of our patients experience recurrent cancer, which is uni-formly fatal. As a result, we often discuss end of life and goals of care as well as other sensitive topics, such as fertility pres-ervation. Discussing end-of-life issues with 75- or 80-year-old women is hard enough, but many elderly patients take their ill-ness in stride by saying, in essence, "Well, I guess I have to die of something." In contrast, discussing death with young women is emotionally taxing for our entire team. Death is the furthest thing from a young person's mind, so they understandably have a hard time switching to a palliative mindset and instead often request more and more treatment even when treatment is no longer helpful.

Strategies for Approaching Sensitive Conversations

Sensitive conversations about goals of care require a great deal of preparation. I focus mostly on curative therapy in the early stages of disease. Our conversations focus on details of diagnos-tic evaluation and treatment, and I repeat the mantra of cure. This process is not that difficult, because we are in our com-fort zone discussing biomedical and logistical information. It is almost as though our patients and we distract ourselves from the prospect of death by busying ourselves with all the details of evaluation and treatment. However, once the cancer recurs, we have to change gears and set realistic expectations for the future. I try to discuss prognosis incrementally over time with each inflection point in their illness, such as when we switch to salvage therapy at first recurrence. One of the most challenging things we do is walking the fine line between offering realistic expectations while not destroying hope. We impress upon patients that we can still help them live better and maybe longer, even if they are incurable.

When patients with recurrent small cell cervical cancer ask me if their condition is curable, I equivocate ever so slightly by saying, "I have been practicing medicine long enough to never say never and never say always, and so I cannot say with 100% certainty that you are incurable. Having said that, cure is extremely unlikely." I am not entirely sure why I equivocate in this way, but I suppose I do so to maintain some degree of hope. The problem with this strategy, however, is that some patients conclude that they will be the one in a million who achieves cure. On the other hand, unrealistic hope may not always be a bad thing and may actually be therapeutic as long as patients continue to make well-informed decisions along the way. As the disease progresses and patients become less and less able to tolerate therapy, my tone shifts from, "You are unlikely to be cured" to "You will not be cured." I approach conversations about goals of care by chipping away a little at each visit and planting seeds so that patients will not feel blindsided at the last moment when they find out we are out of options other than palliative care.

Throughout my career, I have occasionally observed colleagues who do not have incremental, frank conversations with their patients as they pass through different stages of illness in what I think is a misguided attempt to maintain hope. However, this strategy backfires when they suddenly switch to a purely palliative approach, and patients are utterly shocked, reacting as though they had never considered that death was even a distant possibility. I try to have incremental conversations that balance length of survival and quality of life. I usually say something like, "We always want to consider quality and quantity at every step and make sure if we extend your life with treatment, it is a life worth living."

Small cell cervical cancer is exceptionally rare, with only about 200 to 250 cases per year in the United States. As a result, most of my patients hear from their oncologists back home that they have never cared for anyone with small cell cervical cancer, or have only seen one case. Over the past several years, we have established ourselves as an expert referral center. When patients come to us, we develop a definite plan based on our knowledge and experience, unlike their referring doctor, who frequently does not know what to do. We may not be able to cure all our patients yet, but we are equipped to care for them as well as anyone else in the world. We instill confidence in our patients when we tell them that we know how to treat their rare illness. Many patients ask me whether I have ever seen someone with small cell cervical cancer before, after their doctor at home told them they had never seen a single case. I can often honestly tell them that they are the second or third patient with their diagnosis whom I have seen that day. Confidence is contagious.

Tuning into "Scanxiety" and Other Stressors

Patients who are fortunate enough to achieve remission after initial treatment of their small cell cervical cancer experience stress related to "scanxiety," or worrying that their cancer will recur. We routinely get restaging scans the day before surveillance visits, so patients have to wait overnight to hear the results. I can only imagine how excruciating it must be for them to wait and suffer through a sleepless night. As a result, whenever possible, I call patients the night before their appointments to tell them that their scans look fine so they can sleep better. However, this strategy could backfire the next visit if results are not available the day before, because patients may interpret no news as bad news. I therefore make an effort to warn patients that if they do not hear from me the day before, it does not necessarily mean bad news. Sometimes the results do not come across my desk that quickly.

In addition to worrying about recurrent cancer, I think patients are generally much more depressed and anxious than they let on during clinic visits. They seem to put on their best face in front of the doctor, probably to encourage us to continue to aggressive treatment. I know this from personal experience, since my sister-in-law had pancreatic cancer and stayed in our home on and off during the 18 months of her treatment. I accompanied her to clinic visits, and I saw how she would always put on a confident and upbeat face for her oncologist even though she was extremely depressed at home. Most days she would not even get out of bed or eat but when she was at her appointments, she said, "I am a fighter. Nothing will stop me. I am doing great." I think as a profession we could do better at supporting our patients emotionally. Many patients seem to fall through the cracks from the psychosocial standpoint. We probably underemphasize emotional wellness because our training focused more on diseases, but whatever the reasons, we need to do better.

System Approaches to Addressing Psychosocial Distress

Fortunately, in recent years, we have engaged supportive/palliative care much more than we did before. Not long ago we consulted supportive/palliative care primarily to facilitate hospice referral, but now we involve them much earlier in the disease trajectory and with greater frequency. In the future, we also hope to engage members of the psychosocial team to support patients and families who experience the highest levels of distress and establish regular meetings of all members of our clinical team to debrief emotional encounters and to honor patients who die.

Our patients' Facebook group is another powerful source of emotional support. Patients with small cell cervical cancer experience many highs and lows, since they are either celebrating someone's good results together, or more commonly mourning someone's death. Over time the Facebook group has become larger and more cohesive, so about 10 years ago they decided to hold an annual meeting, which first took place in New York City and then in Las Vegas. They actually invited me to the meeting in Vegas, when only about 15–20 women attended. Since then, they have held the meeting every year, and I attend every one. I always take the research staff with me to the annual meetings, because I think it is important for them to see the impact they are having on these women afflicted by the disease. About 100 women and caregivers attended the most recent meeting before the pandemic began, of whom about 35–40 are receiving treatment. Seeing them bond over dinner is one of the highlights of my life. They demonstrate tremendous love and support for one another and even call themselves the "Small Cell Sisters." They have my back, and I have theirs.

The Power of Legacy

As important as psychosocial resources are for the emotional well-being of our patients and our staff, I was on my own as I stood listening to the plaintive cries of my patient in clinic late that afternoon. She was a 36-year-old woman who received chemotherapy for small cell cervical cancer at home but experienced several side effects, after which her cancer quickly recurred. Her oncologist explained that her cancer was incurable and suggested that she focus on quality of life and dignity rather than taking additional treatment. As a single mother of three young children, she thought this option was out of the question. How could she just give up the fight? She traveled to MD Anderson searching for any treatment options, either standard or experimental, since she was still highly functional and otherwise well. A major driving issue for her was that she was divorced from the father of her children and she did not feel that he was fit to care for them. Besides wanting to stay alive for herself and her kids, she did not want them to grow up in his household.

> *When I met my husband, he was such a nice guy. Little did I know he was cheating on me from day one. I knew he liked to party. We even partied together. Oh yeah, he was a lot of fun all right, but he got to the point that he drank all day and then started getting into meth, cocaine, and anything he could get his hands on. We had a nice little house, but all our money went to drugs and booze, so we could not make the mortgage payments.*

I listened silently as idyllic scenes of my childhood home in Malibu flashed before me in sharp contrast to the scenes she described. "*All our money was going to his partying and cheating.*" I imagined how difficult life must be for her as compared to my life, nurtured by parents who were happily married for more than 50 years and now surrounded by a loving wife and children. "*I had to get a second job waiting tables.*" I chuckled slightly to myself as I remembered the story of my dad's patient, the young Hollywood star who no longer needed to wait tables. "*I cannot imagine my kids growing up around him and his women. Who will…?*" I could see she was working herself into a frenzy, so I felt the need to intervene. However, the more she spoke, the less she breathed. She gave me no openings.

I tried to imagine how my father would respond to this desperate young woman. I never saw him speak to a patient in the clinical setting, but I clearly remember the many times I saw him interact with patients who we ran into around town at the grocery store or at restaurants. The thing I remember most is how ecstatic his patients were to see him. If their young children accompanied them, they would literally shove the kids into his arms and glee-fully exclaim, "This is the doctor who brought you into the world!" He did not say much and was shy when he first met people. In fact, some people thought he was a snob before they got to know him well. In reality, he was an incredibly kind person who assumed good intentions, gave people the benefit of the doubt, and treated everyone with respect. He was not the kind of person who took over a room with his effervescent personality at social gatherings but would instead spend time with the people he cared about the most, engaged in meaningful conversation.

I finally interrupted my young patient in mid-sentence. *"I am so sorry to interrupt, but I want to take a brief time out. Is that OK?"* She looked at me quizzically, paused for a moment, and continued her tirade: *"My youngest son hardly knows his father. He gets bad grades in school and still wets his bed…."* I felt the need to refocus her. *"Let's just take a deep breath for a moment, OK?"* She finally paused just long enough for me to continue. *"I can see you are getting increasingly distressed the more you talk, so I want to refocus our conversation on how we can best help you today in the few minutes we have remaining. Would that be OK?"* She looked up through her tears and nodded silently. I imagined what my dad would say and continued:

> *I cannot possibly know how hard your life is. It sounds as though you love your children dearly and want only the best for them. I can tell you are worried about your kids' future after you are gone. I wish I could say something or do something that would make your troubles disappear, or at least help you feel better. I know I cannot fix your problems, but I have a suggestion, anyway. Is it OK if I share my thoughts?*

She seemed a bit surprised by my request but nonetheless nodded yes.

> *Here is what I want you to do before your next clinic visit in a few weeks. You can think of this as a homework*

assignment. I want you to write down all the advice you want to give your children if you die before they grow up to adulthood. You can write down everything on plain paper, in an album, or on a card. It does not matter where you write your thoughts.

Alternatively, you can make a video if you prefer. Tell them all the things you want them to know. For instance, you can tell them how much you love them and how import-ant it is that they live a healthy life and avoid alcohol and drugs. You may want to tell them to treat others with kind-ness. You can also share your hopes and dreams for them.

I recalled my dad's advice whenever I second-guessed or kicked myself about a patient who was experiencing a rocky postoperative course. He would say, *"The only surgeons who do not have complications are those who do not operate. Bad things happen even if you do everything right."* He was telling me to believe in myself. I continued:

You may want to tell you kids to believe in themselves no matter what, to respect everyone, rich or poor, and above all else demand respect from others, since they are worthy of love and respect. Think of yourself as their guardian angel, look-ing down on them, protecting and guiding them after you are gone. Give them something to always remember you by and to cherish forever.

As I spoke, her facial expression transformed from fear, anger, and sadness to steely determination and focus. She had her marching orders. I again thought of my father and the example he set for me. He died five years ago, but he still visits me every day to guide me through my toughest moments, when I am exhausted, frustrated, or scared. He is that little angel on my shoulder.

PRACTICE POINTS

Key Reflections

- Frustration and anger are normal and healthy emotions occasionally experienced by clinicians who care for vulnerable patients with serious illness, especially under emotionally charged circumstances.

- When negative emotions arise, clinicians can adapt by drawing on their inner strength and confidence to regain equilibrium and composure.

- Family members often serve as guiding lights for clinicians to help them navigate life's inevitable challenges and hardships.

- Bad medical outcomes that are beyond the control of the clinical team often happen even if patients receive outstanding care. Great clinicians accept the inevitability of bad outcomes and maintain faith in their skills, compassion, and good intentions.

- Caring for young adults who suffer from grave illness can be extremely emotionally challenging for the healthcare team, especially if those patients have young children and parents who are still involved in their care.

- Many clinicians overemphasize biomedical and technical aspects of care at the expense of emotional and psychosocial aspects. Great medical care is a team sport that requires input from counselors, psychologists, social workers, chaplains, and other members of the psychosocial team.

- Clinicians often benefit from time with colleagues devoted to debriefing emotionally challenging encounters and processing their grief regarding death and other losses.

Empathic Actions

- Great clinicians treat all their patients with the same respect and care, regardless of their socioeconomic status or influence. All patients are special.

- Sometimes showing that we care about a vulnerable patient by simply being present can be even more therapeutic than medical interventions.

- Social media can serve as platforms by which patients and their clinicians support one another emotionally in the face of grief, sadness, or fear.

- Patients with serious illness gain the most from conversations about goals of care and prognosis if they have time to process those conversations incrementally over time.

- One of the most challenging tasks of a great clinician is walking the fine line between offering patients realistic expectations while encouraging them to maintain hope. The key to success is telling patients the truth compassionately.

- Engaging patients in legacy work often helps them take stock of their lives and connect in powerful ways with the people who are most important to them. Such work involves asking patients to reflect on how they want others to remember them, what they hope and dream for their children, what they want to express to others (such as "I love you"), how they want their children to conduct themselves after they are gone, and other open-ended exploratory questions that encourage reflection.

Empathic Expression

- I can see you are getting increasingly distressed the more you talk, so I want to refocus our conversation on how we can best help you today in the few minutes we have remaining. Would that be OK?

- I cannot possibly know how hard your life is.

- It sounds as though you love your children dearly and want only the best for them. I can tell you are worried about your kids' future after you are gone.

- I wish I could say something or do something that would make your troubles disappear, or at least help you feel better. I know I cannot fix your problems, but I have a suggestion, anyway. Is it OK if I share my thoughts?

17 A Brief Clinician's Guide to Empathic Expression

Laura G. Meyer and Daniel E. Epner

Understanding Empathy

Empathy can be thought of as standing in the patient's shoes or trying to imagine the patient's perspective. Empathy involves reframing the clinical encounter by recognizing emotion and occupying the emotional space rather than defaulting to a biomedical or factual stance.

How to Use This Guide

This guide provides a brief conceptual framework for empathy in patient care and provides examples of difficult situations or phrases and suggested responses. Each vignette is a mere snapshot of situations that commonly arise in medical practice. We propose "traditional" responses in the left column and "empathic" responses in the right column.

Guide Layout	
Traditional Approach	**Empathic or Exploratory Approach**
Difficult patient encounter as depicted by scenario or "patient quote."	
An example of a traditional response to the scenario by the provider.	An example of the preferred empathic response by the provider.

All clinicians should adapt the responses in this guide to their own style and use words and phrases that feel genuine to them. "Traditional" approaches listed in this document are often appropriate in the right context.

Empathy in Patient Care: *Key Concepts*

KEY CONCEPT 1: The challenging conversations described in this guide are born of strong emotions that are experienced by all vulnerable patients and their families. Those emotions include fear, helplessness, desperation, frustration, sadness, grief, and anxiety.

KEY CONCEPT 2: Rather than trying to fix the unfixable, empathic responses like those listed in this guide help us to connect with patients and families in a healing way.

KEY CONCEPT 3: Exploratory questions, like, "tell me more…," create more empathic opportunities.

KEY CONCEPT 4: Empathic responses often fit into one of the following categories (**NURSE**): **N**ame the emotion, **U**nderstand, **R**espect, **S**upport, **E**xplore (Pollak, *Journal of Clinical Oncology* 2007).

Examples of Empathic Continuer Statements to Stimulate Expression	
Name (the emotion)	I can imagine you are feeling sad/nervous/angry…
Understand (validate)	I can/can't imagine… …how difficult this must be for you and your family. …how you're feeling. I don't blame you for feeling…
Respect	I respect your: • fighting spirit. • love for your family. • courage. • strong faith. Faith is powerful medicine. • independence. • resilience.
Support	We will be here for you throughout this process no matter what happens. You are not alone.
Explore	Tell me more… • about what you meant when you said… • about how you and your family are coping…
I wish…	…things were different. …we had better treatments for you. …I could fully relieve your symptoms…

Weaving Empathy into Every Encounter

Traditional Approach	Empathic or Exploratory Approach
Scenario: On the way to the patient's room, you see him in the hallway on his way to the cafeteria.	
"Would you mind going back to your room now? I would like to find out how you are doing."	"I'm glad to see you out and about. We will circle back to you later when you're back in your room. Have a good lunch!"
You enter the room and notice an empty bed, but a family member is in the room.	
"Oops! I thought Mr. Y was here. I'll come back later."	Provider: "Hi! I'm Dr. X from the supportive care team here to see Mr. Y. His primary team asked us to help relieve whatever symptoms he has. How are you related?" "I am his wife." Provider: "It's nice to meet you. I will come back a little later to speak to both of you."
Entering the room	
"May I come in? (patient grants permission) I am Dr. X from supportive care. Your primary team asked us to help you with your pain and other symptoms. Will you please fill out this symptom inventory? I will be back in a few minutes."	"May I come in? (patient grants permission, but doctor notices patient is eating) I am Dr. X from supportive care. I see you're eating. Would you like me to come back later?" Or "May I come in? (patient grants permission but appears subdued) I am Dr. X from supportive care. You look really tired/quiet/sad. Tell me what's on your mind."

(Large support network present)	
"I am Dr. X from supportive care. Your primary team asked us to help you with your pain. Where do you hurt?"	"I see you have several visitors today. How is everyone related?" Or "Wow, you have so many visitors here with you today! You are quite popular."

Collecting Data Empathically

Traditional Approach	Empathic or Exploratory Approach
Edmonton Symptom Assessment System (ESAS)	
"I'm going to run through a list of symptoms, and I need you to rate each of them on a scale of 0–10 (0 being none, 10 being the worst you could possibly imagine). How would you rate your pain?"	"We've already talked about your pain, but I want to ask you about a few other symptoms, if that's OK with you. I know this is a lot of work, but may I ask you to rate these other symptoms from 0–10?"
Memorial Delirium Assessment Scale (MDAS)	
"I have some silly questions that we ask everybody every day. What is today's date?"	Provider: "The pain medicines you're on can often make people foggy, so I want to ask you a few questions to check your mental clarity. Would that be OK?" Patient chuckles nervously and says: "I'm not so sure about that, but go ahead, I guess." Provider: "It's OK if you don't know the answers to all the questions. I just want to see if the medications need to be adjusted." *(Start with the easiest questions and progressively move to more difficult questions.)*

CAGE Substance Use Screening Tool/Screener and Opioid Assessment for Patients with Pain (SOAPP)	
Provider: "Have you ever felt guilty about the amount of alcohol you consume or had to take an eye-opener first thing in the morning?" Patient: "Oh not this crap again. I'm not a drug abuser." Provider: "We ask these questions for your safety."	Provider: "Have you ever felt guilty about the amount of alcohol you consume or had to take an eye-opener first thing in the morning?" Patient: "Oh not this crap again. I'm not a drug abuser." Provider: "I know answering these questions repeatedly can be frustrating and annoying, but it's really important that we get this information so we can provide you the best and safest care."

"Denial"

Key Concept: When patients and their families have an unrealistic or overly optimistic outlook about prognosis, clinicians often conclude they are "in denial." This disconnect is born of strong emotions, including grief, fear, sadness, frustration, desperation, and anxiety. Clinicians should therefore respond with empathy.

Traditional Approach	Empathic or Exploratory Approach
"We're not ready for hospice."	
"Hospice is really great. They will attend to your comfort and quality of life and help you live as well as possible."	Provider: "People have a lot of different expectations. Tell me more about what you understand about hospice." Patient: "My aunt was in hospice, and all they did was give her morphine. She was dead in a day!" Provider: "It must have been hard to see her like that. This is a big change for you, and I know it must be scary."

"I can't stop life support. This is my daughter. I can't give up on her."	
"I hate to see her suffering like this. She has no realistic chance of recovery."	"I can see how much you love your daughter and can't bear the thought of losing her. I respect how hard you're fighting for her. It must be hard to see her like this."

"We want our mother to be alert and talk to us like she did just the other day."	
"I don't think I can keep her comfortable and alert at the same time. She will get agitated if I lower the dose of pain medicine."	"I can tell that you love your mom and want what is best for her. I can also tell that you desperately want to maintain your connection to her. What would you tell her if she were more awake?"

"I don't want to be at the mercy of drugs, I just want to be normal again."	
"These medications are the best shot we have at keeping you as comfortable as possible and maintaining your quality of life."	Provider: "Tell me more about what you mean by 'normal.'" Patient: "I want to get stronger and return to work. I am not giving up." Provider: "This must be a huge change for you. I am afraid this may be a strong as you get. I wish we could do more to help you gain strength."

"They told me no more treatment, but I'm a fighter, I will get stronger so I can start more treatment."	
"We're going to help you get stronger so you can start more treatment." (false hope)	"I respect your fighting spirit." Or "I'm afraid this may be as strong as you get." Or "What would be most important to you if you are unable to get stronger?"
"He was walking a week ago and playing golf. He's going to get better."	
"This is how the disease progresses. It's part of the process."	"It must be hard to see him like this." Or "I can imagine these changes must be shocking."

"I don't care what the doctors say. What do I have to lose by taking more treatment?"
Key Concept: Sometimes a dose of reality using a traditional, factual approach is the best strategy.   "You have a lot to lose, including your dignity. Additional treatment will almost certainly harm you and increase your suffering rather than help you."

"I have faith God has a plan for me. I am sure I will be completely healed."	
"We can always hope for a miracle."	"I admire your strong faith. Faith is powerful medicine."

"Do you believe in miracles?"	
"Yes, but, if God is going heal you, he will do so with or without artificial support."	"Tell me more about what you mean by 'miracle.'" Patient: "I mean being cured and fully restored to health." "That is a wonderful dream. I only wish we could make that dream a reality. I wish it were that simple. Have you thought about how you would want to live if you don't achieve a miracle cure?"
"I don't want to talk about machines or DNR, but that's all you people want to talk about. I'm not ready for that."	
"We just want to do what's best for you to maintain your quality of life."	"I know it can be really hard to talk about such serious topics, and I know you've been inundated with all this bad news. Many people who are as sick as you are like to hope for the best but still plan for the worst. However, it sounds like you are not ready to discuss worst-case scenarios."
"You're going to just let me die?"	
"This is the natural process of cancer progression. We want to help you maintain your quality of life. Treating the cancer at this point will harm you."	"I know it must feel that way. I wish we could do more to help you. I promise that no matter what happens, you are not alone. We will help you any way possible."

"I don't want him to go to the palliative care unit, because he won't get the same care there as he does here."

"We can't do any more for him on this unit. These nurses are outstanding, but they focus more on the cancer than on quality of life, which is our main focus now."	"I can only imagine that moving away from this unit can be very scary, because the nurses and the rest of the team here know you so well. Tell me more about the types of care you still hope to receive."

Provider: "I understand Dr. X mentioned the Palliative Care Unit to you. What are your thoughts?"
Patient: "Dr. X never said anything about moving. I'm not giving up! I want more treatment."

"I'm sorry about the confusion. I can ask Dr. X to come back by to speak with you so we're all on the same page."	Provider: "I can imagine how shocked you feel hearing this from me, especially because you're just now meeting me for the first time. Tell me more about what Dr. X told you about your options." Patient: "She told me if I get stronger and gain weight, I can enter a clinical trial." Provider: "We can always hope for improvement, but I'm concerned this may be as strong as you get. Regardless of what happens, we will support you any way we can. I will also speak to Dr. X to make sure we are on the same page."

"I know he is brain dead and there's nothing more you can do for him. Stop telling me that."	
"I'm terribly sorry for your loss."	"I'm terribly sorry for your loss. I can tell you need some time with your son to honor him and say goodbye. I will come back to check on you a little later. Do you need support from the chaplain or counselor? Is there someone else you want at your side now?"
"I want to be full code now." (Code reversal)	
"CPR will be very traumatic for you and your family. For instance, chest compressions will probably break your ribs, which will be painful and undignified."	Provider: "Tell me more about this decision." Patient: "My daughter just got here from California, and she told me I shouldn't give up. I was playing tennis just a few weeks ago! I want to see my grandkids again." Provider: "It must be really shocking for your daughter to see how your condition has changed since she last saw you. I respect the fact that she is fighting for you. What do you think she knows about your condition? Do you think we can meet with her when she visits you?"

Prognosis

Traditional Approach	Empathic or Exploratory Approach
"How much time do you think I have?"	
"It could be as soon as today, although I think you have days to weeks."	"It could be as soon as today, although I think you have days to weeks. It is very hard for us to estimate accurately. Not knowing can be the hardest part. Tell me more about why you ask about life span. Help me answer the question the best way possible."

"Why can't you cure him?"	
"He hasn't responded to treatment the way we'd hoped."	"I wish we could do more for him. We are trying desperately to develop better treatments for cancer, but we have a long way to go."
"Will I ever be normal again?"	
"I think so. Let's see how things go."	Provider: "What do you mean by 'normal'?" Patient: "Hike in the mountains and kayak like I used to, return to full-time work, and play with my grandkids." Provider: "It sounds like you have always taken good care of yourself and have lived life to the fullest. I can't say how you will feel after surgery, but you will probably have to adjust to a new normal. Regardless of the outcome, we will help you maintain the best quality of life possible every step of the way."
"I'm in Supportive Care Clinic today because my oncologist told me that if I get stronger and gain some weight, I can get more chemotherapy."	
"Ok. We will refer you to physical therapy and a dietician to help you meet those goals."	"We can always hope for you to get a lot stronger, but I'm concerned this may be as strong as you get. Have you ever thought about what will be most important to you if you cannot take chemotherapy?"

"I can't believe I have cancer. I take good care of myself: I've never smoked, done drugs, or drank alcohol. I eat well and exercise."	
"Sometimes cancer develops for no particular reason."	"I know this comes as a shock to you. This cancer is certainly not your fault. Sometimes bad things happen to good people for no reason."

Existential Concerns

Traditional Approach	Empathic or Exploratory Approach
"Doc, I'm ready for this to be over. Help me end this now. I want you to help me die."	
"You know there are laws against euthanasia in Texas." Or "We can't hasten your death intentionally, but we want to help you live better."	Provider: "I can't imagine how much pain you've experienced through this process. I can tell you are ready for this ordeal to be over." Patient: "I am done. I've had it!" Provider: "Is there anything you want to tell people or tell them again at this point, like how much you love them? Would you like to work with our psychosocial team to create legacy documents, such as letters or videos for your loved ones to see after you die?" Or "Tell me more about what you are most proud of in your life, or how you want to be remembered."

"I'm not sure what there is to look forward to. What's the point of trying anymore?"	
"I'm concerned you may be depressed. Have you ever taken an antidepressant?"	"You've been fighting your cancer for so long. It sounds like you're fed up with this whole ordeal. Is there anything else you want to accomplish in your life?"
Patient in "total surrender," unwilling to engage in communication.	
"We will come back later when you are in the mood to talk. We will also send our counselor by."	"It seems like you are completely worn out. I can only imagine how difficult it is to have so many people coming in to talk to you, especially about such serious news. Is there anything I can do for you now?"
"I can't believe God would abandon me like this."	
"God never abandons us, but he sometimes works in mysterious ways"	"It sounds like you have a strong faith, but that you are beginning to question God's plan after all you've been through." "Yes, I don't deserve any of this. I never drank, smoked, or took drugs. I have always taken care of my body, and now I end up like this: a bag of bones." "I don't blame you for being angry. None of this is your fault."
"I have two kids and two step-kids, but I haven't spoken to them in years. They sometimes call me on Christmas."	
"We can ask our social worker to help you contact them on the phone."	"It sounds like you've had some rough times along the way. It must be difficult not to be able to speak with your kids and see them regularly."
"I guess I shouldn't be surprised I got cancer. I smoked like a chimney for years."	
"Smoking does cause cancer."	"You're being really hard on yourself. No one is perfect."

"Where am I going after this?"	
"That is the ultimate mystery."	Provider: "Wondering about what happens after death can be very scary. Would you like to meet with a chaplain or your own spiritual leader?" Patient: "No, I am not the religious type." Provider: "Tell me more about what worries you the most."

"You can't possibly understand how I feel. I'm dying, and I'm only 36! You are perfectly healthy. Don't try to convince me to feel better with your psychological mumbo jumbo."	
"Talking to a counselor when you're feeling this depressed can be helpful."	"You're right – I can't imagine how you feel. It must be annoying to hear people tell you how to think or feel, on top of everything else. We will support you to the best of our ability and adapt to your preferences."

"I am receiving this new treatment and I know I will be cured. I do not need to discuss anything else at this point."	
"Ok."	"I can imagine it must be incredibly hard to talk about serious news over and over. We will remain available to meet in the future if you want."

"It's not that I am being negative, but how can I live the life I want when I can't do anything anymore. I am in bed all day in pain. What kind of life is that? I don't think anyone would want to live this way."	
"Let us try to help you feel better. I really think we can help you."	"I can only imagine how difficult this is for you."

"Why are you taking away my hope?"	
"We never give up hope. We hope you will have the best quality of life possible."	Provider: "I am sure when we talk about such serious news over and over it seems like we are taking away your hope. What do you hope for at this point?" Patient: "To become normal again. To be completely cured." Provider: "That would be so wonderful if you were cured and back to your normal self. I would love to see that. What are some other things you hope for if you are not cured?"

Family Impact

Traditional Approach	Empathic or Exploratory Approach
"I don't want to talk to my kids about this. I need to be strong for them."	
"We have counselors who can talk to you about having these conversations with your children."	"I can see how much you love and want to fight for them. How much do you think they already know?"
"I'm worried about how much this is costing them." Or "I feel like a burden on my family."	
"You've helped them all these years. I'm sure they will be happy to help you now."	"You've always been the one to take care of everyone else. It sounds like you did a great job raising your kids." Or "I can't imagine how difficult it is to be the one who needs help now."

"I moved into my son's house when I got sick so he could help take care of me. He takes time off from his job to take me to my appointments. I enjoy seeing my grandkids every day."	
"I'm sure he doesn't mind taking care of you."	Provider: "I can see how important your family is to you. It sounds like you have done a great job raising them." Patient: "I don't feel like the same person anymore. My son does so much for me. I feel like a burden." Provider: "I can only imagine how hard it is for you to depend on others when you've been the provider your whole life."
"What will happen to my kids? My family needs me."	
"I'm sure someone in your family will step up. Let's focus on you."	Provider: "Tell me more about your concerns." Patient: "I worry about them, like, who's going to take them to school, who's going to cheer for them at soccer, that sort of thing." Provider: "It must be scary to think about not being there for them. I can see that you care deeply for them. Would you like to meet with one of our psychosocial team to discuss this further?"
"What if I'm not there for my daughter's sixth birthday?"	
"Let's try to get you stronger."	"That must be a really scary thought. (pause as patient cries) I can see how much you love her and can't stand the thought of not being here for her. Provider (after patient settles down): Have you considered doing legacy work?"

"I want to be able to walk her down the aisle. Can you make that happen?"	
"We'll do our best."	"I can see how important it is for you to be there for your daughter on such a big occasion. I'm concerned this is as strong as you will get. Do you want to talk about how to celebrate her wedding even if you can't walk her down the aisle?"
"Will my children remember me?"	
"I am sure they will. You shouldn't worry about that, because you must have many pictures they can admire as they grow up. Your memory will live on forever in their hearts."	Provider: "Tell me more about your children. How old are they?" Patient: "My son is 3 and my daughter is 8 months old." Provider: "The thought of not being here for them as they grow up must be heart-wrenching for you. I dearly wish we could cure your cancer. However, under these circumstances, many people find it helpful to do legacy work. Do you know what I mean by legacy work? Would you like to meet with a counselor to learn more about it?"

Difficult Family Dynamics: Directing Empathy Towards Family Members

Traditional Approach	Empathic or Exploratory Approach
"Dad, you can't give up! You have to see your grandkids grow up."	
"Your father isn't giving up. He's fighting for his quality of life and dignity."	"I can see how much you love your dad, and I respect how hard you are fighting for him. It must be brutal for you to see him like this. I know you have had great times together."

"I hate when you talk about giving up. We're not quitters in this family. You always told me never to quit."

"Your father isn't giving up. He's fighting for his quality of life and dignity."	"It sounds like your dad has instilled a true fighting spirit in you and has set a great example. You are a true warrior, and I respect the fact that you risked your life overseas to protect our freedom. I also know your dad is no quitter, because I, like you, have seen how hard he has fought this illness. He is tough as nails, and so are you."

"Oh, it doesn't matter what he thinks. He may be the sick one, but we make his decisions for him."

"I realize you are his medical power of attorney, but we have to make sure to respect his wishes. Did he complete an advanced directive before he became incapacitated?"	Provider: "What do you think he would want if he could speak to us?" Family member: "He would want to cure his cancer or at least fight it until the end." Provider: "What else would be important to him in addition to curing his cancer?" Family member: "He always said he never wanted to be a vegetable on a machine at the end of life. He told me he wants to go in peace when his time comes."

"I know my daughter is suffering greatly, but she said, 'Never give up on me.' I have to honor her wishes, so I can't make her DNR."

"When I put on this white coat several years ago, I promised above all to do no harm, and I mean to honor that promise."	"I can see how much you love your daughter and I respect how hard you're fighting for her. I can only imagine how painful it is to think of life without her. Tell me more about what you mean by 'giving up.'"

"Please don't tell my mother she has cancer or any other bad news."	
"We have to tell her about her disease in order to offer her evaluation and treatment."	Provider: "Tell me more about your concerns and why you don't want us to tell your mother." Patient's son: "I'm concerned that she will give up all hope and stop fighting." Provider: "I respect how hard you're fighting to protect your mother. You obviously love her a great deal. You have traveled so far to get here; you carry a heavy burden on your shoulders."

Anger or Hostility

Traditional Approach	Empathic or Exploratory Approach
"My mother and I came all this way because this is a world-famous cancer center, and you're telling me there's nothing more you can do for her?"	
"We're certainly going to do everything in our power to find better options."	"I respect how hard you are fighting for your mother's welfare. It must be really difficult to be so far away from home, especially when you're not getting the news you hoped for." Or "I wish we had better options for your mother. I promise to do our best by her no matter what."
"You're 45 minutes late. You're treating me like I don't matter!"	
Key Concept: Apologize when appropriate. "I'm so sorry to keep you waiting. You must be hungry by now. A patient in another room had an urgent medical issue that I had to attend to, but now you have my full attention. Would you like us to get you a snack?"	
"This place has failed me miserably."	
Key Concept: Empathize rather than debating or being defensive. "I don't blame you for being angry. I wish we could do more for you."	

"Of course I'm depressed! Wouldn't you be if you were told you are going to die?"	
"Have you ever taken an antidepressant?" Or "I hate to ask such a sensitive question, but have you considered taking your own life?"	"It must be incredibly difficult to hear such serious news. I can't imagine…."
Family member: "You can't understand how painful it is to outlive your own child. Do you have children?" Provider: "Yes." Family member: "I hope *you* never experience losing one of them."	
"I hope so too."	"You're right, I can't possibly understand how devastating it must be to lose a child. I can only imagine."

Suspected Nonmedical Opiate Use or Unusually High Pain Expression

Traditional Approach	Empathic or Exploratory Approach
"Doc, I know where you're going with this. I hate to be asked all these questions all the time. You're talking to me like I'm a criminal and you think I'm trying to sell my pain medicines."	
"We're doing all this for your safety and the safety of those around you."	"I hear you're frustrated. I know it's hard to hear these questions repeatedly, but we want to make sure you're using your pain medications safely and getting the most benefit from them. I get really worried when you can't accurately describe how you use your meds and you sometimes take them in ways that are different than how we prescribe them."

"You don't know how I feel. I may not look like I'm hurting, but I have a high pain tolerance. I need meds."	
"I'm just trying to do what's best for you now."	"I can't possibly know how you feel. I realize you are suffering. Our job is to follow safe practice to help you live as well as possible."
"I've been coming to this clinic for two years, and every doctor has given me the meds I need. You are the first doctor who has denied me."	
Key Concept: Oftentimes, empathy should be tempered with a dose of reality. "Your situation now is different than it was before. I know it seems like I'm being punitive, but I really just want to take good care of you and make sure we use these medications safely."	
"I am afraid I will become addicted."	
"Do you or anyone in your family have a history of substance use?"	Provider: "I can see why you're nervous about that. Tell me more about what worries you." Patient: "My daughter is addicted to dope and has been in jail a few times. I finally had to break off ties with her. I'm raising her two-year-old daughter." Provider: "It sounds like you're going through a real rough patch. It must be hard to see your daughter suffer like that, and I'm sure you're suffering too."
"I've been giving my son some of my pain medication."	
"You should not share your medications, and your son should take only what we prescribe him in the way we prescribe it."	"I can understand why you would, because you can't stand to see him suffering like this. If he were my kid, I might do the same thing. I can tell you really love him and will do anything for him. Having said that, I think we can do an even better job taking care of his symptoms, and we think it's important that you not share medications with him for everyone's safety."

"Weed is the only thing that helps. I smoke five times a day."	
"Marijuana is illegal and unregulated. We don't want you to mix the marijuana with the pain medications."	"I don't blame you for doing everything you can to get by. Cancer is not easy. Having said that, I think we can do a better job of controlling your symptoms than you can with marijuana. In addition, I'm concerned marijuana won't mix well with your other medications, like pain medication."
"I got this weed from a state where it's legal, so it is regulated."	
"It's not regulated in Texas, which is where we are. Therefore, I cannot and will not recommend using it."	"I don't have any moral stance on using marijuana, and I realize it's legal in many states. However, I'm concerned about potential side effects between marijuana and your other medicines like your pain medicines. We want to work with you to try to taper off marijuana to the extent possible."

Universal Themes

Traditional Approach	**Empathic or Exploratory Approach**
"I'm scared."	
"Many people are here to support you." Or "Do you take medication for anxiety?"	Provider: "Tell me what scares you the most." Patient: "I'm scared of dying." Provider: "Thinking about the unknown is scary. Tell me more about what scares you about dying." And "Would you like to meet with a chaplain or other spiritual leader?"

"I can't even look in a mirror now. I'm so depressed."	
"Have you ever taken an antidepressant?" Or "I hate to ask such a sensitive question, but have you considered taking your own life?"	"It's normal for people to be concerned about their body image when they go through such arduous treatment. Have the changes in your body kept you from doing social activities like going out to eat or visiting with friends? Have the changes in your body affected your relationship with your husband?" And "The changes in your body are not your fault, and anyone would be upset under these circumstances. I know before your illness you took great care of yourself and exercised and ate well. These changes must be shocking. I can't imagine how hard this is for you. Would you like to discuss these issues with a counselor?"
"Will I be in pain like this forever?"	
"No, of course not. We can't completely eliminate your pain, but we can adjust your medications and help you feel much better."	"That must be a scary thought. I think we can help you feel much better by adjusting your medications."
"I'm afraid I will suffer in the end."	
"Our job is to make sure that you suffer as little as possible."	Provider: "Tell me more about what you're most concerned about." Patient: "I'm afraid I'm going to suffocate. I'm already short of breath." Provider: "That must be a really scary thought. We will make sure to give you medications to relieve the sensation of breathlessness. We will help you no matter what."

Index